A Brush with Cancer

10 Years of Sharing, Connecting, and Healing

TWIST® OUT CANCER

A BRUSH WITH CANCER: 10 YEARS OF SHARING, CONNECTING, AND HEALING

EDITORIAL
Joshua Taustein, *Editor-in-Chief*
Lindsay Patton, *Features Editor*

DESIGN
Jeff Guerrero, *Creative Director*
Giorgia Lupi, *Featured Artist*

PUBLISHER
IngramSpark

CONTRIBUTING PHOTOGRAPHERS
Alison Conklin
Aleya Cydney
Liesl Diesel
J & J Photography
Einav and Amit Payes
Shelby Ricci
Louis Terry

CONTRIBUTING WRITERS
Soraya Fata
Anna Feneis
Jenna Koch
Lindsay Patton
Jenna Benn Shersher
August Spree
Joshua Taustein

EDITORS
Mardi Kaplan
Kenny Lapins
Lindsay Patton
Jenna Benn Shersher

CONTRIBUTING INSPIRATIONS
Aliza Ainis
Jenna Benn Shersher
Fayruz Benyousef
Jonelle Binder
Kathleen Brown
Kristina and Jim Burke
Briana Camilleri
Virginia Champoux
Colleen Connelly
Pam Crowther
Theresa Daly
Soraya Fata
Grace Fauls Lombardo
Jeffrey Froggett
Raychel Funk
Carol Garrett
Lisa Glick
Joni Goldstein
Staci Greenfield
Jackie Herigodt
Tiffany Horstein
Kirsten Johnson
Mardi Kaplan
Sonya Keshwani
Debbie Lubeck
Roger Joseph Mommaerts, Jr.
Kim Kass
Bob Kaufman
Jennifer King
Devon Messner
Noah Plotkin
Arielle Prichard
Rachel Reichblum
Eyal Schecter
Jamie Schmidt
Sharon Seeder
Maya Shany
August Spree
Karen Tabascio
Bobbie Tiedt Donohew
Kathryn Tubbs
Sarah Wartell
Dr. Michael Weiner
Danielle Williams
Rena Williams
Matthew Wolniewicz
Vital Zinger

CONTRIBUTING ARTISTS
Judy Abplanalp
Tish Amparan Daniel
Lauri Andreacchio
Dr. Sharon Arffa
Ishita Banerjee
Nissim Ben Aderet
Amanda Bodie Stenlund
Melissa Burgess
Taurus Burns
Jacqueline Carmody
Renee Chase
Murielle Cohen
Dr. Collin Reiff
Jenny Conlee-Drizos
JD Dennison
Mignon Dupepe
Anna Feneis
Sujata Gazder
Nicole Gordon
Erin Greganti
Akiva Gross
Jeff Guerrero
Ofer Katz
Michele Kellner
Shefali Khanna
Bowen Kline
Bryan and Liz Kuntz
Kenny Lapins
Taylor Lazzara
Maura Matthews
Dr. Ruth Mayer
Marie McGrory
Tony Nguyen
Jennifer O'Brien
Thomas Pyrzewski
Kirk Roda
Nancy Rosen
John Stumbaugh
Joey Tea
Kara Thomas
Kathryn Tubbs
Kate Van Doren
Amanda Walker
Brad Young

Find Us Online
www.twistoutcancer.org

ONLINE RETAIL STORE
www.shoptwistoutcancer.org

FOLLOW US
@twistoutcancer

This book is dedicated to those that have bravely chosen to come forward with their story and have resisted the desire to retreat from fear. It is their tenacity and resilience that have built this beautiful community. And to the artists who have given so much of themselves to support our inspirations, we are forever grateful for your generosity.

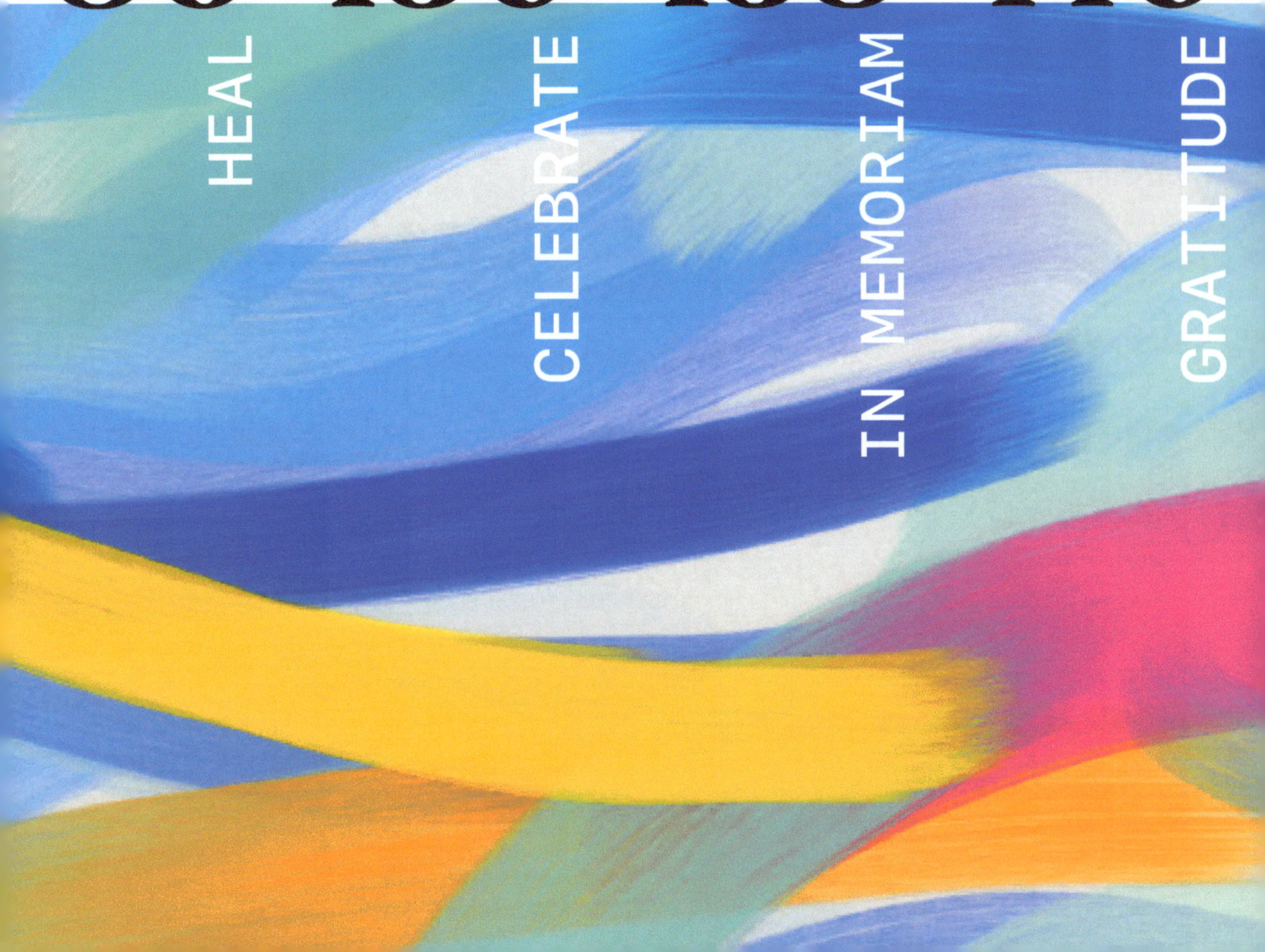

A Note from Jenna

While it is now an organization filled with and driven by love and compassion, Twist Out Cancer was born from a desperate and lonely place.

When I was 29 years old, I was diagnosed with Grey Zone Lymphoma, a rare blood cancer, which at the time, impacted fewer than 300 people worldwide.

As a young adult facing a rare type of cancer, doubts, fears, and questions of why and what will happen were threatening to be my constant, weary companions if I didn't dig deep and seek meaning in my suffering.

Fighting a rare type of cancer as a young person throws your hopes and dreams into a state of delirium. Plans stopped. Aspirations deferred. As my life story became distilled into a series of cherished moments, time was no longer my own. My life as I knew it was on hold.

As I learned to exist in this holding pattern, I started to notice that young adults with cancer had a unique set of needs that were not being met and certainly were not being talked about. Who could we share this grief with? Without release, it surely would consume us faster than the dreaded disease we were fighting.

When we don't speak about what's hard, we feel shame. It was the shame that tried to paralyze me, but instead inspired me.

I found myself revisiting one of my favorite authors, Viktor Frankl, a psychiatrist who survived the Nazi death camps and has imparted incredible wisdom and lessons on survivorship.

One statement in particular resonated with me:

In 'Man's Search for Meaning,' Viktor Frankl said "Everything can be taken from a man but one thing: the last of the human freedom—-to choose one's attitude in any given set of circumstances, to choose one's own way."

How can we change our attitude when things are TRULY hard? I chose to Twist Out Cancer.

Twisting Out Cancer means seeing my crisis as an opportunity, choosing to turn a hardship, a diagnosis, a disease, into a chance to help others. I knew that I could take the darkness and reflect back the light of sharing and empathy.

I needed to accept the situation I was in to come up with a plan to manage it. Once I embraced it, I was able to see it as an opportunity for growth not only for me but for others around me.

Twisting Out Cancer means Sharing Big Dreams. When I was diagnosed with cancer, I knew that I would be fighting not only for my own life, but also for my chance to one day bring life into the world. From that dream, I drew power. What dream will your crisis propel you to reach for? The best time to dream big is when you have nothing left to lose. It provides a filter by which we can assess the ties that bind us. It empowers us to embrace only those connections essential to our wellbeing, only those that feed us love and companionship.

Twist Out Cancer means Connecting. Enduring a crisis can be lonely. It is critical to connect with others who get it. Maybe I could create a safe space where others could find their crisis soulmate, someone to whom they can open up and begin to heal the spaces that neither chemotherapy nor radiation can reach. I wanted to help people to build their squad by choosing wisely among others who could commiserate and celebrate.

Twist Out Cancer means Healing Ourselves and Others. When we have found those with whom we want to share our journey, we hold onto them fiercely. The universe is big, and to travel it without support and love is a dark prospect. Sharing our fears, sharing our triumphs, sharing our loves is what life is about, as it turns out. Twist Out Cancer is about helping those who have been tried and tested and connecting them with others who are on the same path. And when those who want to share find connection with those who want to receive, everyone heals. From the darkness, there is light. From despair, there is hope. From sadness, there is love.

When I look back on this incredible journey over the last 10 years, I am struck by the mystery of it all. Out of the depths of a terrifying diagnosis blossomed a beautiful gift. Now, Twist Out Cancer has foundations deeper and more sound than the disease that inspired it. It shines as an example of how the indefatigable human spirit can find strength in adversity. To all of the people who have joined this mission to bring psychosocial support to those in need and bring beautiful art into the world, thank you. Each day that passes, each event that we put on, each canvas that gets painted, is another victory, another step toward the day when all of this is no longer needed. In the meantime, here's to the next 10 years of sharing, connecting, and healing.

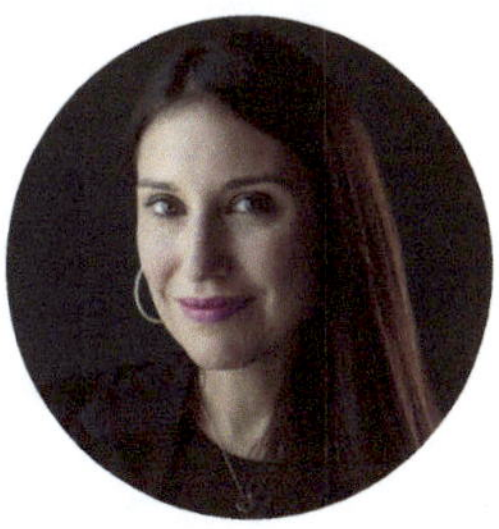

With love and gratitude,

Jenna Benn Shersher

Jenna Benn Shersher

Founder and CEO of Twist Out Cancer

Little Pieces of Twist-ory

Celebrating 10 years of any sort is a huge feat, but it took a village, lots of love, and dedication to grow Twist. Here's a look at how we got to where we are today.

2012
Jenna founded Twist Out Cancer out of her apartment in Chicago. It started with a staff of one and 12 dedicated Board of Directors.

2013
The first Brushes With Cancer program launched at Floating World Gallery in Chicago, featuring 20 Inspirations and 20 Artists.

2017
For the first time, two Brushes With Cancer programs were held in the same year - in Toronto and Chicago.

2018
The Brushes With Cancer program expanded internationally, holding programs in Montreal and Tel Aviv.

2019
Hosted programs for the first time in Detroit, Philadelphia, and Austin. The year wrapped up with a sold out gala at Moonlight Studios in Chicago.

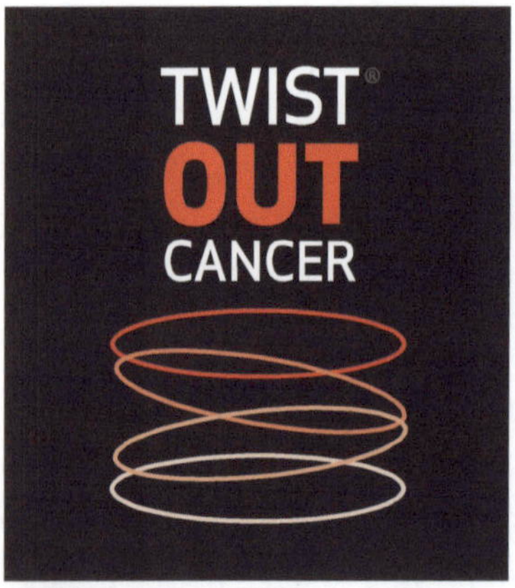

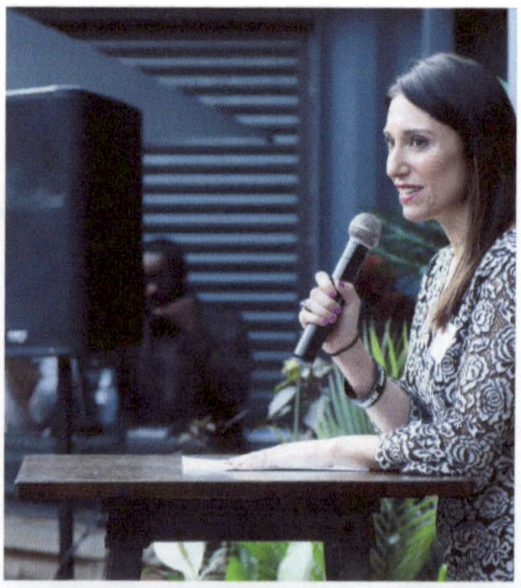

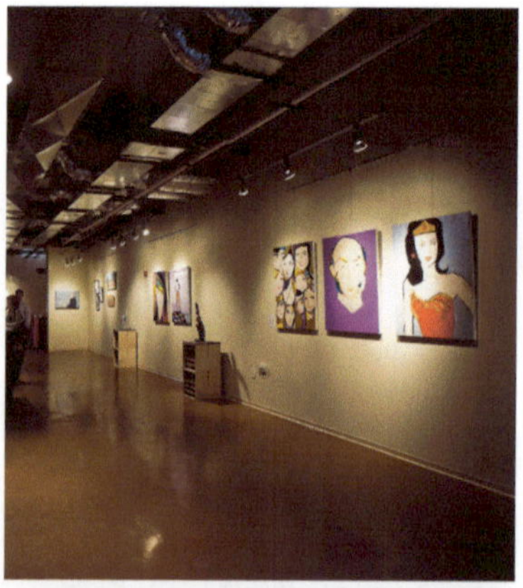

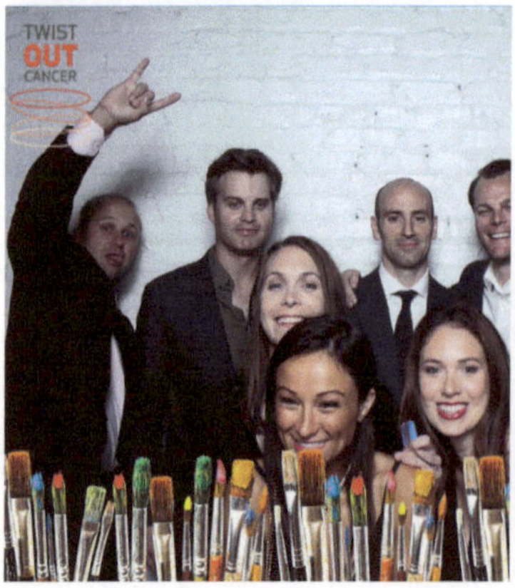

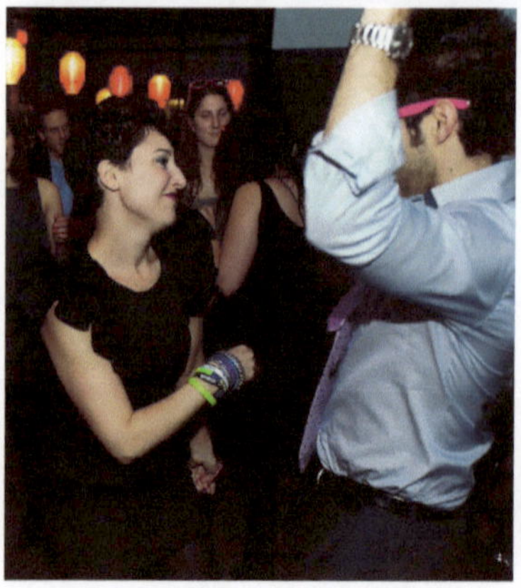

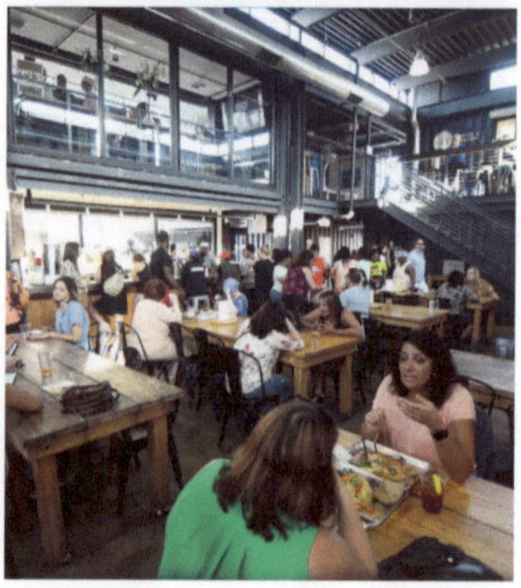

2014
The second Brushes With Cancer program was held in Chicago, featuring 22 artists and 22 inspirations.

2015
Working with the Canadian Board of Directors, a Brushes with Cancer program was held in Toronto, as well as in Ann Arbor at the Voices Gallery.

2016
A Brushes With Cancer program was held in Chicago with over 750 attendees—our largest year.

2020
Brushes With Cancer went virtual in Austin and Chicago due to the pandemic. Twist received national recognition in the *New York Times*.

2021
The Lancet Haematology chronicled Jenna's journey from a survivor of Gray Zone Lymphoma to a healer as the founder of Twist Out Cancer.

2022
Brushes with Cancer galas held in Austin and Chicago. We'll celebrate our 10 year anniversary with an exhibition at the WNDR Museum in Chicago.

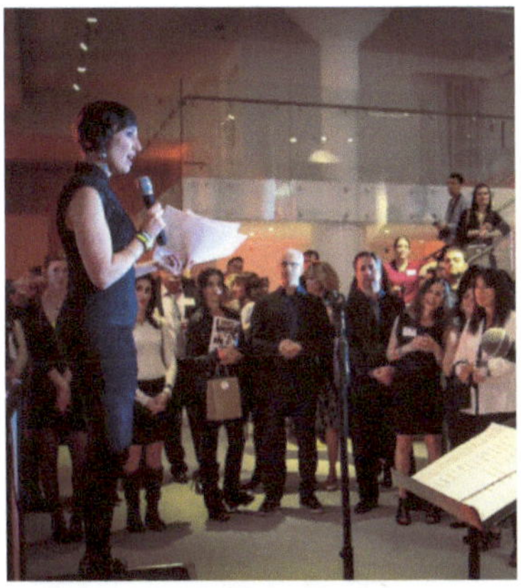

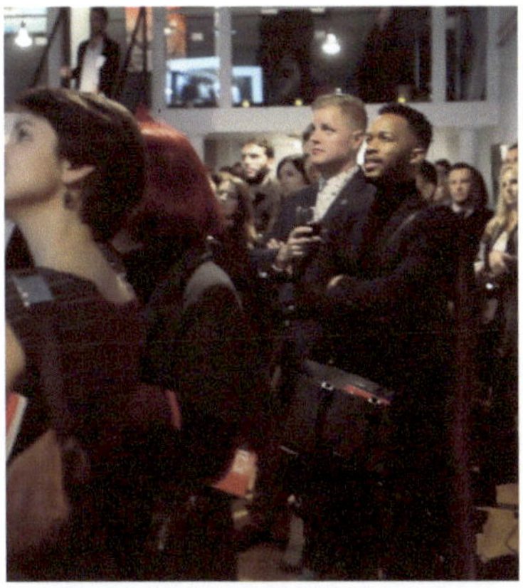

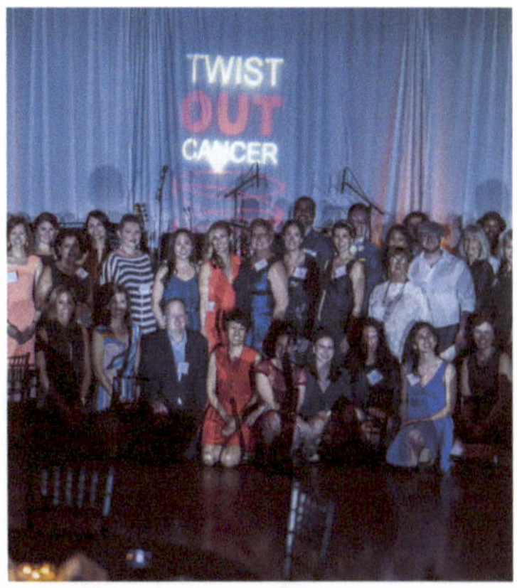

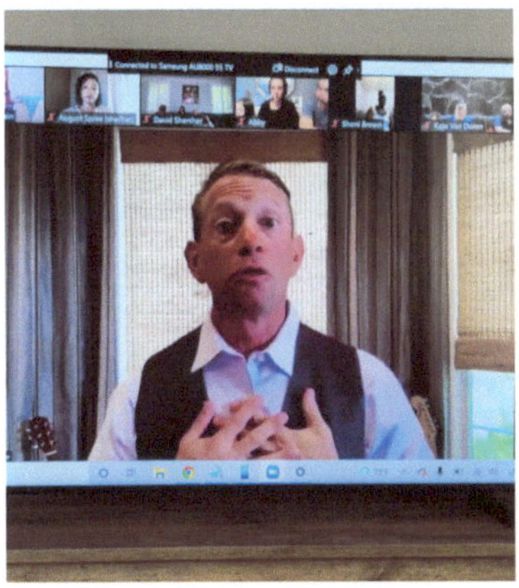

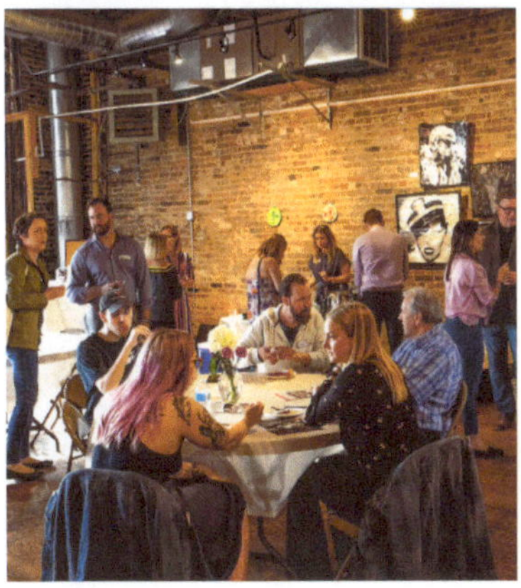

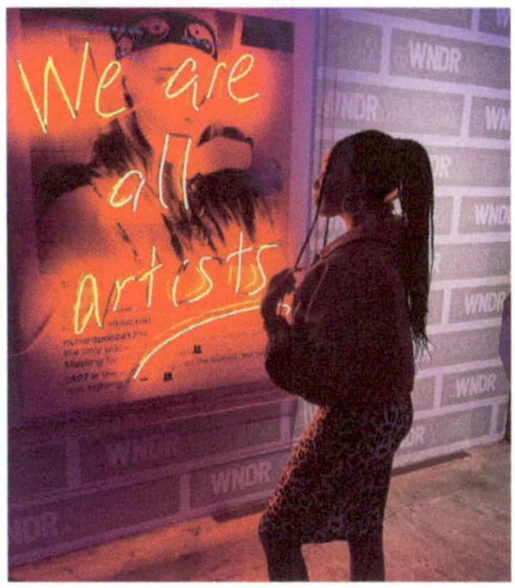

Twist
x
Pentagram

For the last 6 months, Giorgia Lupi and the team at **Pentagram**, a multi-disciplinary design studio, have taken a deep dive into Twist Out Cancer's program, Brushes with Cancer. Enclosed is a visual representation of the intersection between illness and health, art and science, the individual and community, and the profound power of connection.

Brushes With Cancer

Over the course of ten years, Twist Out Cancer has connected over 600 survivors, previvors, caregivers, and artists who have been touched by cancer.

The following page features 278 brushstrokes, which represent the collaborations between these individuals. Weaving in and out of each other, the design shows the deep connections between the Twist Out Cancer community.

Designed by Giorgia Lupi (Pentagram)

How to read it

Each brushstroke represents a person. Their roles are color-coded as follows:

Artists

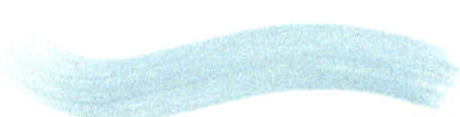

Inspirations

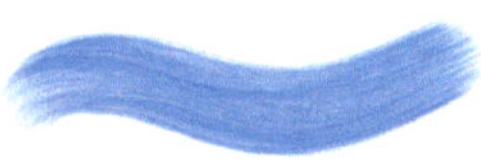

Survivor

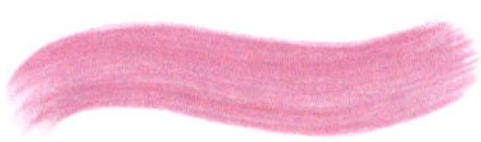

Previvor

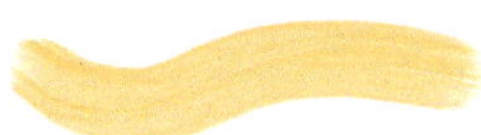

Caregiver

Each collaboration is represented as connected brushstrokes:

As an artist, Alison worked with two inspirations, April and Denise.

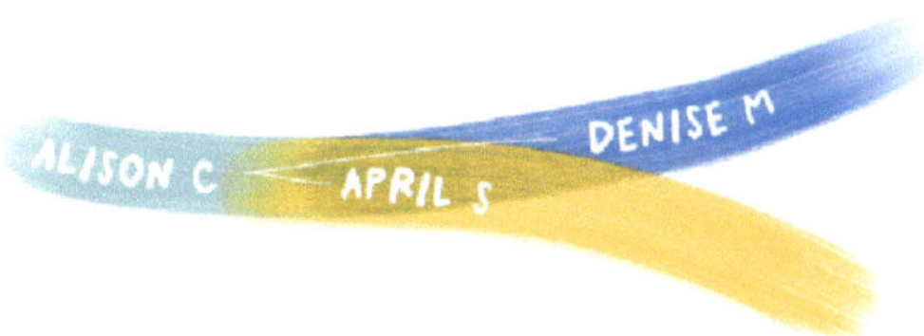

Debbie worked with two artists, Rachel and Amanda.

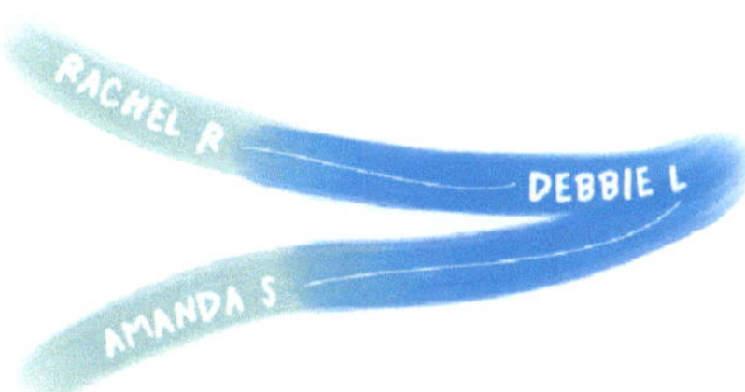

Noah worked as an inspiration with Mignon and as an artist with Jaime.

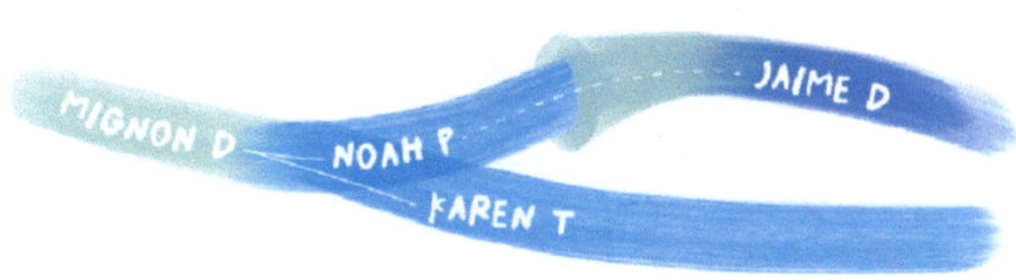

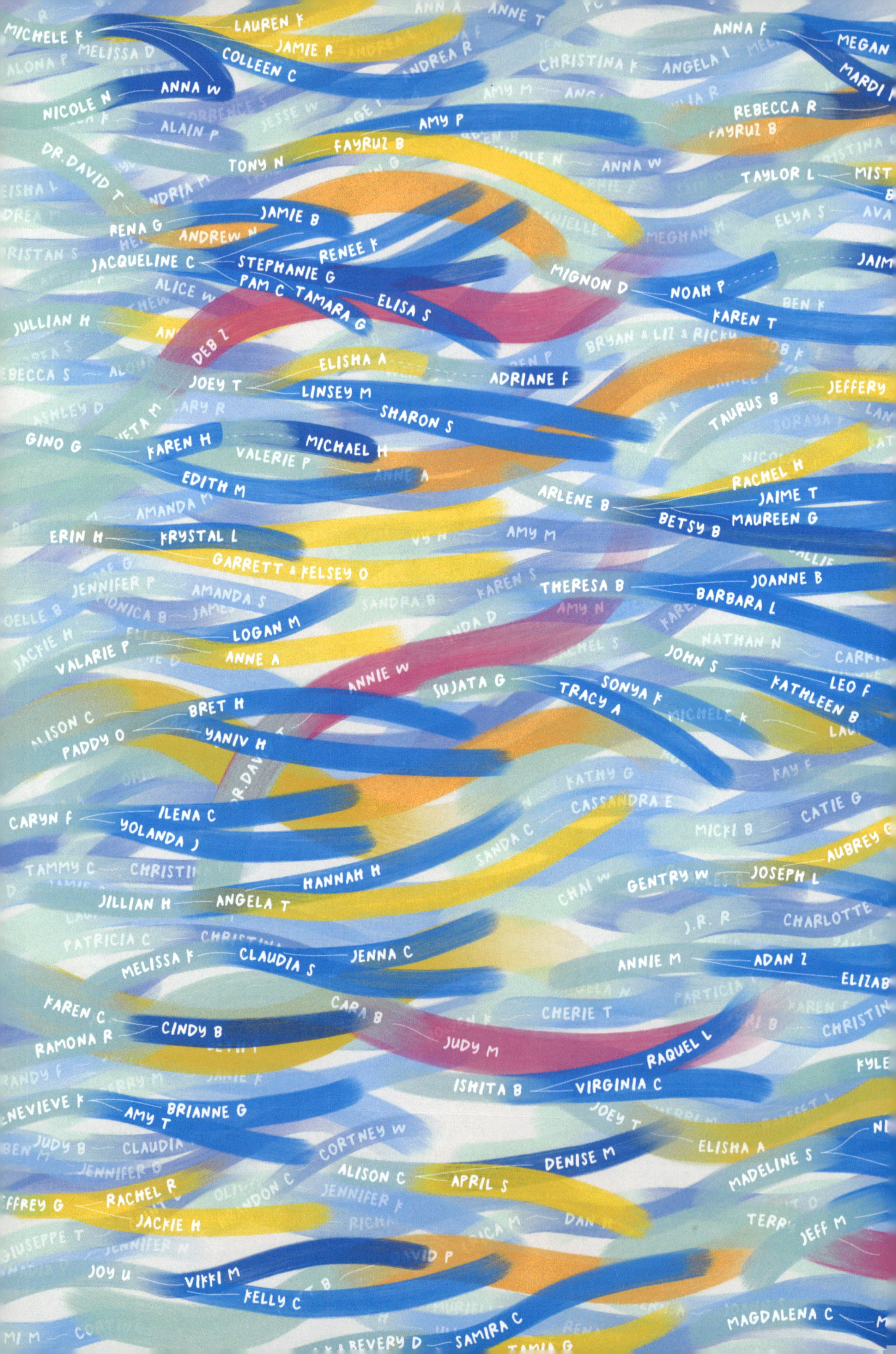

MICHELE K
LAUREN K
JAMIE R
COLLEEN C
ANDREA R
ANNA F
MEGAN
MARDI
CHRISTINA K
ANGELA I
NICOLE N
ANNA W
ALAIN P
AMY P
REBECCA R
FAYRUZ B
TONY N
ANNA W
TAYLOR L
DR. DAVID T
JAMIE B
RENA G
ANDREW N
RENEE K
JACQUELINE C
STEPHANIE G
PAM C
TAMARA G
ELISA S
MIGNON D
NOAH P
KAREN T
JULLIAN H
DEB Z
ELISHA A
ADRIANE F
JOEY T
LINSEY M
SHARON S
TAURUS B
JEFFERY
GINO G
KAREN H
MICHAEL H
VALERIE P
EDITH M
RACHEL H
JAIME T
ARLENE B
BETSY B
MAUREEN G
ERIN H
KRYSTAL L
AMY M
GARRETT & KELSEY O
THERESA B
JOANNE B
BARBARA L
LOGAN M
VALARIE P
ANNE A
JOHN S
ANNIE W
SUJATA G
SONYA K
TRACY A
LEO F
KATHLEEN B
BRET H
PADDY O
YANIV H
CARYN F
ILENA C
YOLANDA J
CASSANDRA E
CATIE G
MICKI B
AUBREY G
HANNAH H
GENTRY W
JOSEPH L
JILLIAN H
ANGELA T
CHARLOTTE
MELISSA K
CLAUDIA S
JENNA C
ANNIE M
ADAN Z
KAREN C
CINDY B
RAMONA R
CARA B
JUDY M
CHERIE T
RAQUEL L
ISHITA B
VIRGINIA C
BRIANNE G
AMY T
CORTNEY W
DENISE M
ELISHA A
ALISON C
APRIL S
MADELINE S
RACHEL R
JACKIE H
JEFF M
JOY U
VIKKI M
KELLY C
SAMIRA C
MAGDALENA C

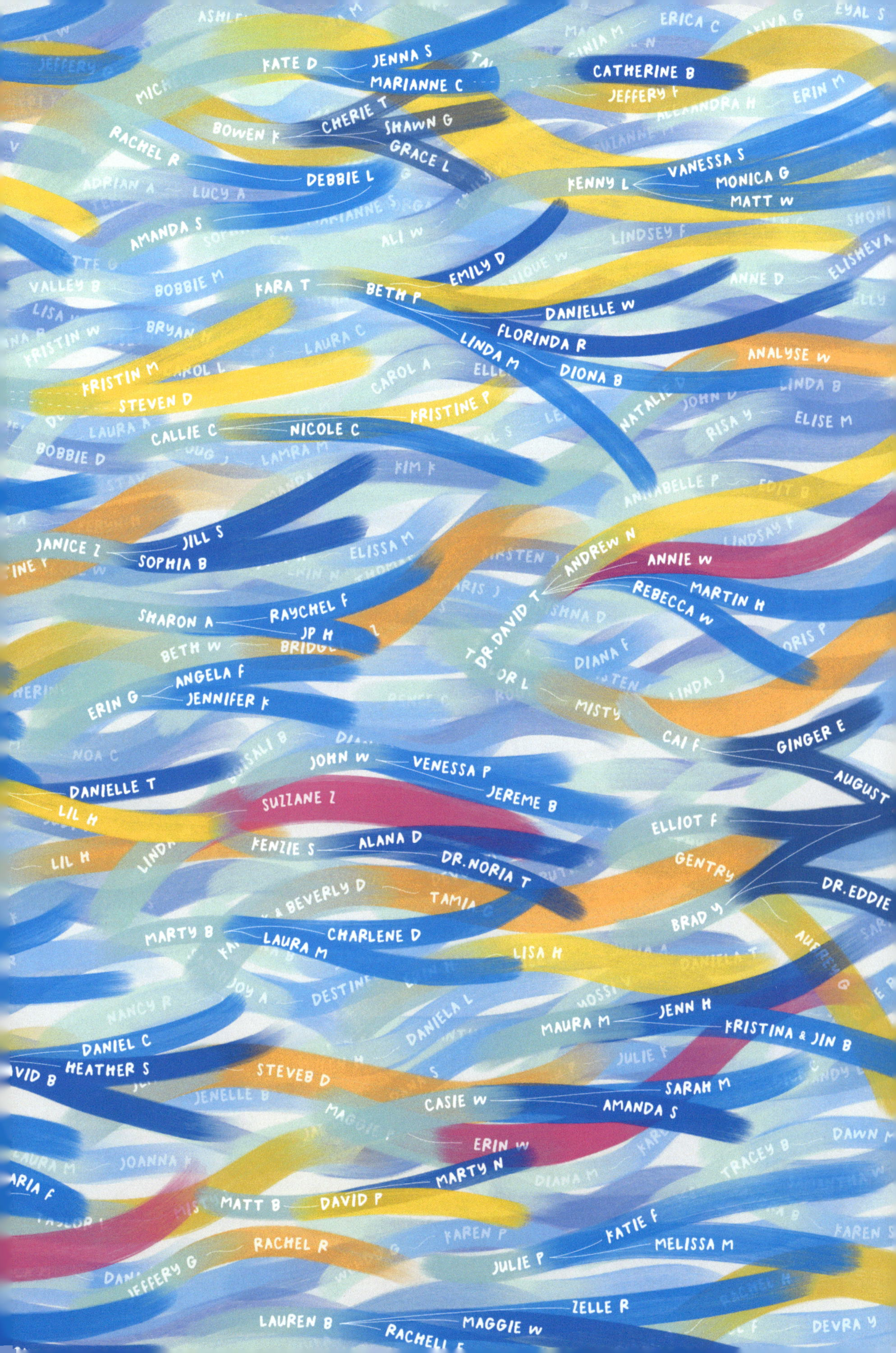

KATE D
JENNA S
MARIANNE C
CATHERINE B
JEFFERY F
ERICA C
EYAL S
ERIN M
BOWEN F
CHERIE T
SHAWN G
GRACE L
RACHEL R
DEBBIE L
FENNY L
VANESSA S
MONICA G
MATT W
ADRIAN A
LUCY A
AMANDA S
ALI W
LINDSEY F
VALLEY B
BOBBIE M
KARA T
BETH P
EMILY D
ANNE D
ELISHEVA
DANIELLE W
FLORINDA R
LINDA M
DIONA B
KRISTIN W
BRYAN
LAURA C
ANALYSE W
KRISTIN M
STEVEN D
CAROL A
KRISTINE P
NATALIE
LINDA B
RISA Y
ELISE M
CALLIE C
NICOLE C
LAURA A
BOBBIE D
LAMRA M
KIM F
ANNABELLE P
JANICE Z
JILL S
SOPHIA B
ELISSA M
LINDSAY F
ANDREW N
ANNIE W
DR. DAVID T
MARTIN H
REBECCA W
SHARON A
RAYCHEL F
JP H
BETH W
DIANA F
ANGELA F
ERIN G
JENNIFER K
MISTY
LINDA J
CAI F
GINGER E
NOA C
JOHN W
VENESSA P
JEREME B
DANIELLE T
AUGUST
LIL H
SUZZANE Z
ELLIOT F
LIL H
KENZIE S
ALANA D
DR. NORIA T
GENTRY
BEVERLY D
TAMIA
DR. EDDIE
BRAD Y
MARTY B
LAURA M
CHARLENE D
LISA H
JOY A
NANCY R
DESTINE
DANIELA L
MAURA M
JENN H
KRISTINA & JIN B
DANIEL C
HEATHER S
STEVEB D
JULIE F
SARAH M
JENELLE B
CASIE W
AMANDA S
ERIN W
DAWN M
JOANNA
TRACEY B
MARTY N
DIANA M
MATT B
DAVID P
KAREN P
KATIE F
MELISSA M
KAREN S
RACHEL R
JULIE P
JEFFERY G
ZELLE R
LAUREN B
MAGGIE W
DEVRA Y

I LEARNED MANY LESSONS AL
MENTALLY AND PHYSICALLY
OVERWHELMING HUMAN K
AND MYSELF, AND PRACTICE
INFORMED DECISIONS WITH

ALTHOUGH CANCER IS THE ONE THING I HATE IN THIS WORLD, IT HAS SHOWN ME A SIDE OF MY FAMILY AND MYSELF THAT I WOULD HAVE NEVER KNOWN WITHOUT THIS TERRIBLE DISEASE. OUR NEW PERSPECTIVE ON LIFE WAS MY DAD'S FINAL GIFT TO US, WE ARE BETTER BECAUSE OF HIM AND FOR HIM.

THAT TAKING CARE OF SOMEONE YOU LOVE WITH CANCER CAN
AND SOUL SO ITS INCREDIBLY IMPORTANT TO HEAL THAT PAI
TO PREVENT CANCER - OR OUTRUN IT AS I OFTEN FEEL IS EXHA
DEBILITATING AS WELL. I THINK THAT WE CAN OFTEN FEEL
EXHAUSTED BY WHAT IT TAKES TO TRY AND ATTEMPT PREVE

OF TAKING SOMETHING FEARFUL, DARK AND PAINFUL AND TURNING IT INTO SOMETHING PRECIOUS. IT IS A TESTAMENT OF GRATITUDE FOR THE FREEDOM, FRIENDSHIPS AND COMMUNITY THAT WAS DISCOVERED THROUGH THE SIMPLE AND BOLD USE OF A SINGLE WORD.

I AM HO
TO SEE HOW
SO DIFFI
MEMORY O
MISS HIM
OTHERS IMP
TRIBUTE T

EVERYTHING CAN LOOK DIFFERENT IF YOU DIVE DEEP ENOUGH. A SECOND GLANCE, A MORE INVOLVED PERSPECTIVE. WE EACH BRING OUR WHOLE LIVES INTO CALCULATING WHAT WE ARE WITNESSING IN THAT VERY MOMENT.

LIVE LIFE IN THE MOMENT. ONLY FOCUS ON THE ESSENTIALS OF LIFE IN REGARDS TO FRIENDS, FAMILY AND WORK. KEEP IT SIMPLE AND NEVER QUIT.

CANCER HAS TAUGHT ME TO BE VULNERABLE, AND THAT IS WHEN I HAVE CONNECTED THE MOST WITH PEOPLE. MY MOST MEANINGFUL RELATIONSHIPS AND CONVERSATIONS IN LIFE HAVE BEEN THE RESULT OF BEING VULNERABLE AND ACKNOWLEDGING THE WORST EXPERIENCE OF MY LIFE.

CANCER THROWS YOU INTO A NEW LIFE. FIRST INTO THE GREY UNKNOWN FOGGY WATER, CHANGING YOU, CHANGING YOUR FAMILY. ITS MUCH LIKE A DEATH WHICH FORCES YOU INTO A NEW LIFE, A NEW WAY OF BEING, A NEW WAY OF BREATHING, A NEW WAY OF LIVING, A NEW WAY OF LOVING.

TRUST IS THE ABILITY TO HAVE CONFIDENCE AND RELY ON THE STRENGTH OF SOMEONE OR SOMETHING OUTSIDE OF YOUR CONTROL. THE CAPACITY TO TRUST IN THE UNKNOWN IS EXTREMELY DIFFICULT WHEN THE REST OF YOUR WORLD SEEMS TO BE IN CHAOS.

AFTER MY BRUSH WITH CANCER, I BECAME
EMOTIONAL AND PHYSICAL WELL-BEING. THROU
I FOUND GROWTH AND A NEW APPROACH TO OUR DA

…ay. I discovered how
…at I am. I experienced
…ward my family
…make difficult, yet
…o poise.

…our heart
…t trying
… can be
…t also
…cer.

This journey taught me to celebrate every moment. I've stopped worrying about what people think and just focused on spending quality time with my family and enjoying every moment. Life handed her the biggest lemon and she has been making the sweetest lemonade ever since.

My experience with cancer taught me to live my life to the fullest. I often worry about the small issues that come along, but always remind myself that I have overcome much bigger hurdles, and that this one is nothing compared to it.

The many "layers" of life experiences that affect us do not make up our being. I believe at our core lies a spirit. That spirit is impenetrable, and we don't know what it looks like. The layers of life do not define us, our spirit does. I encased the piece in resin to make it permanent like the spirit.

…have been part of this program. It is inspiring
…o so beautiful can come out of something
…e part in this project to honour the
…er. He passed away two years ago and I
…o be able to share this experience with
…cancer was a way to help pay
…onderful and courageous man.

Our fight for recovery had failed and our hearts are broken, but we have gained a promise of something positive, an inspiration that I don't have the words to describe just yet.

The three sections of this peice reflect the three times in her life in which her health took control of her life. She powered through each one and never acted as a victim. This piece allows her to have the opportunity for others to listen to her story.

I received one of the most unexpected gift: the strength that can only come by just holding hands and challenging the unknown. For 19 months we fought the inevitable. The balloon popped; the train came charging; we all went down together.

Time is a steering wheel in front of you and it's constantly spinning. Sending you in circles of endless motion. It's menacing, as you wonder if it will ever stop. When cancer hit me, time was un-phased.

…aware of my
…ent and healing,
…spirit…

share.

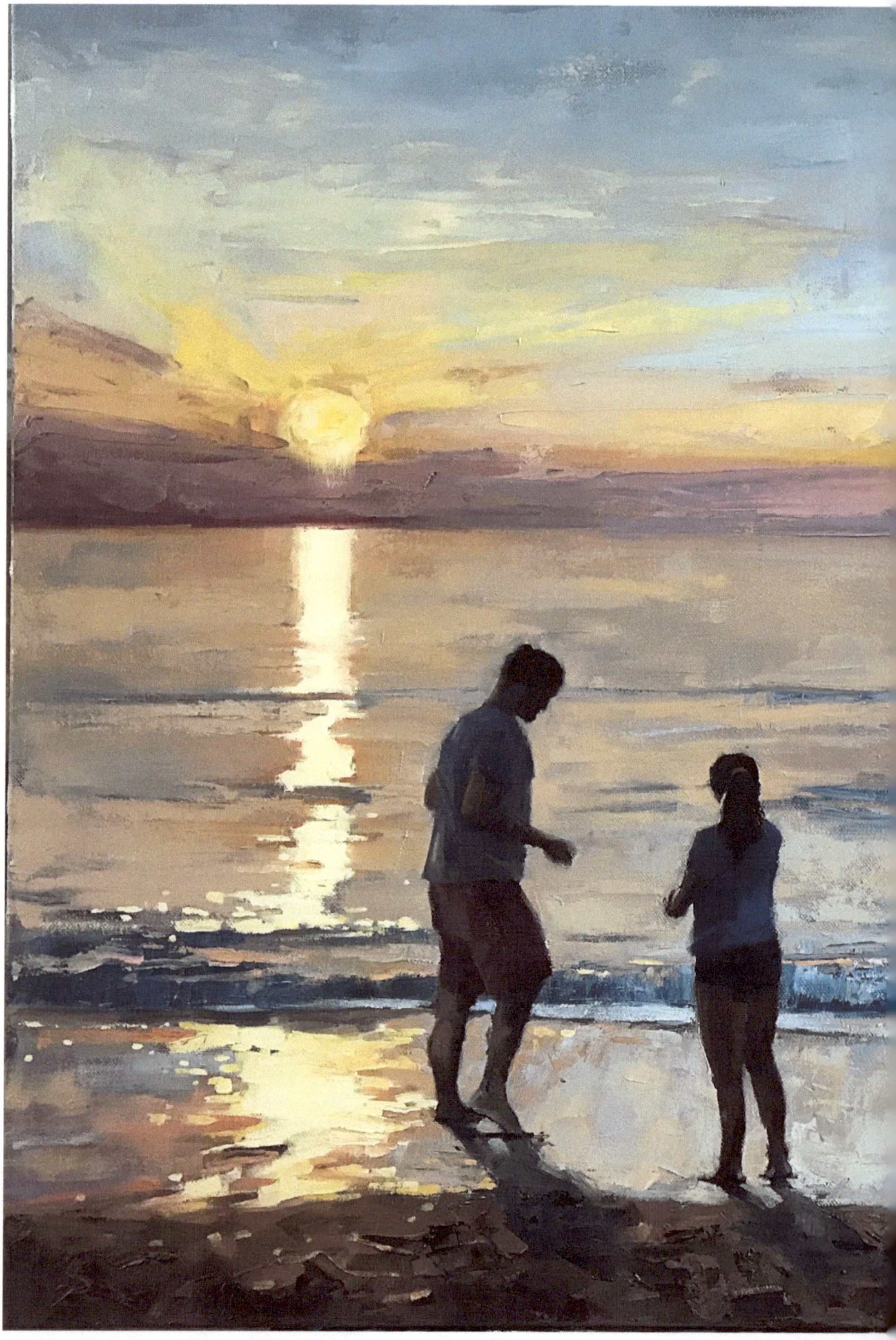

"All Her Ducks in a Row"

Inspiration: Debbie Lubeck
Artist: Amanda Brodie Stenlund

BWC Chicago, 2020

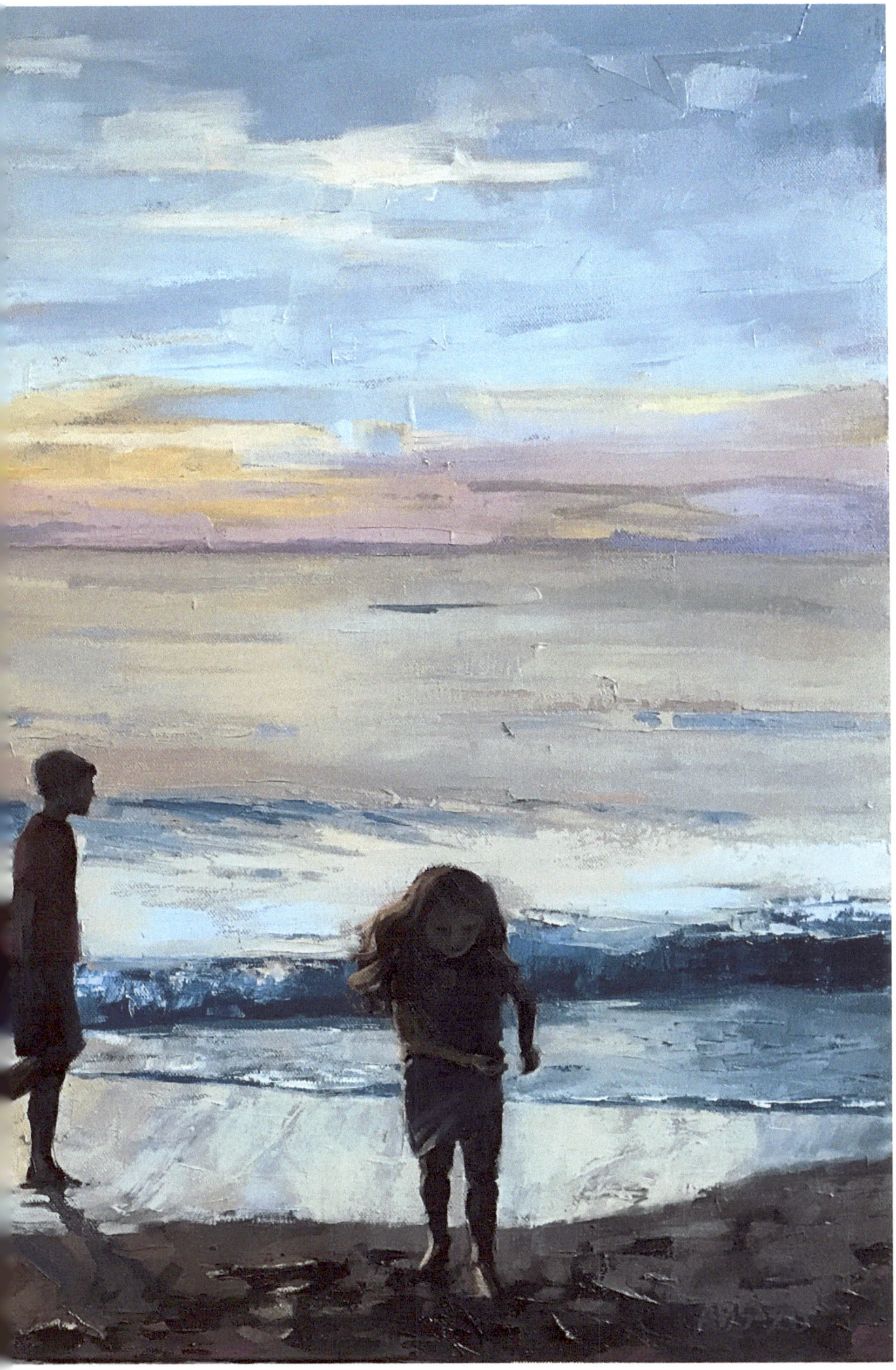

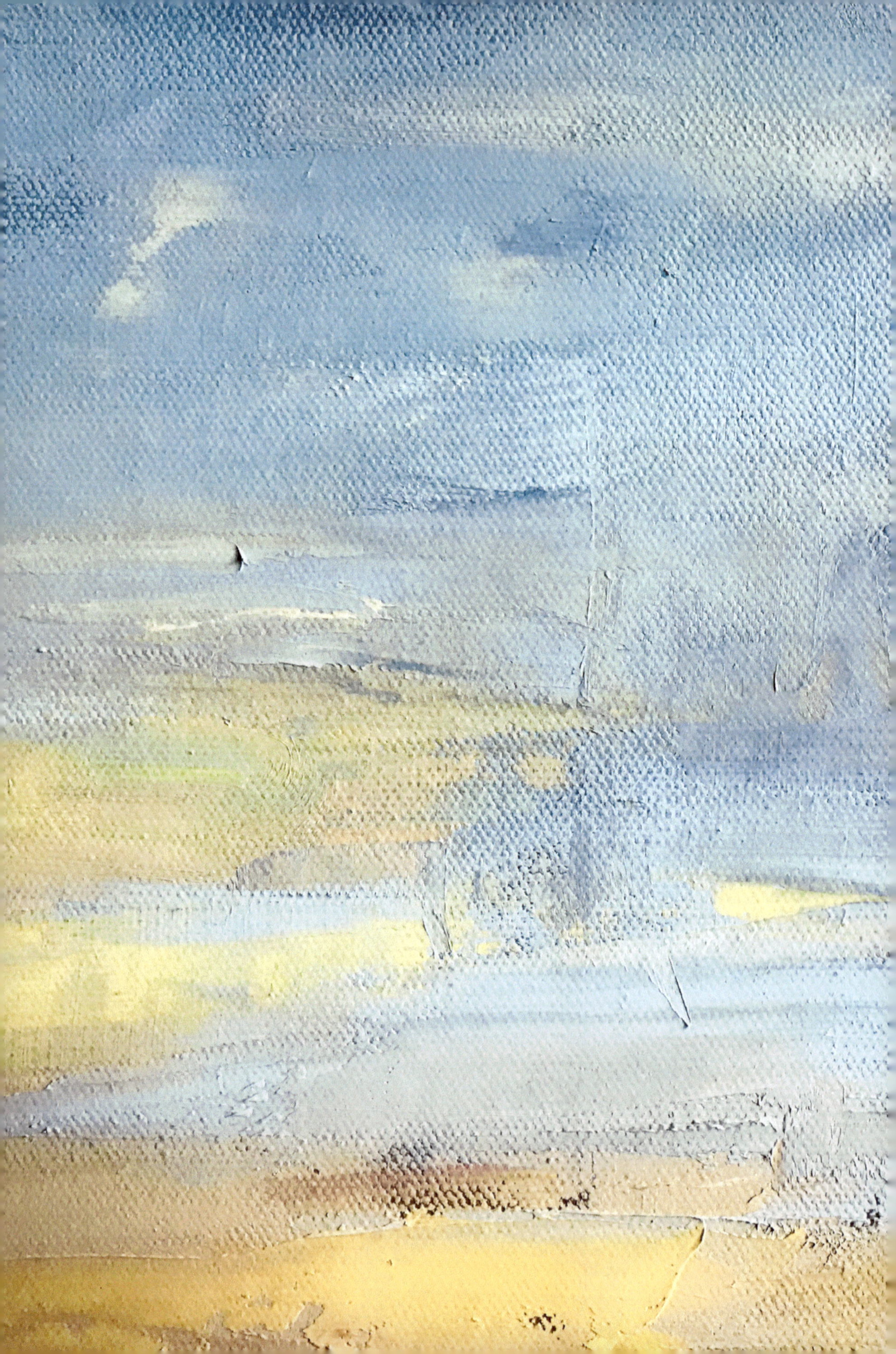

All Her Ducks in a Row

To Debbie Lubeck's children, cancer was a normal part of life. And that's how she wanted it to be for them.

"I put a lot of my focus into protecting the kids and maintaining normalcy," she said. "Clearly, our lives were not normal during any of that, but I didn't want them to know how abnormal it was."

Debbie's situation, though, was extremely abnormal. She was 40 years old and 23 weeks pregnant with her third child when she was diagnosed with breast cancer.

"I was the first pregnant person my oncologist had treated."

As a 2020 Brushes with Cancer Inspiration, Debbie was paired with Artist Amanda Brodie Stenlund. Being similar ages and both having young children, there was a lot to connect on.

"Kids turn to moms for comfort. Moms are their safe place," Amanda said. "Debbie was going to do everything she could to keep being that safe place for her kids, and that is what we have in common."

Of course, those deep, interpersonal connections strengthen over time, which is how Debbie and Amanda's relationship progressed.

"The first few phone calls were like being on a date with someone and getting to know them," Amanda said.

"It was awkward, it's always awkward," Debbie added.

"I'm sure I had a giant glass of rose," Amanda said with a laugh.

But those early, awkward interactions were intentional, and paved the way for an incredible experience for both Inspiration and Artist.

"The thing that struck me with Debbie's story – and what I wanted to focus on with the artwork – was how she was trying to protect her children's day-to-day life from her own day-to-day struggles and fears and stresses with cancer," Amanda said.

While Debbie admitted she was nervous to see the final result, those nerves didn't last long during the reveal.

"It was clear in the finished piece that it was made lovingly – not just paint on a canvas because there was an assignment to do," Debbie said. "It was this moment of, 'Those are my people.'"

Following CDC guidelines, Debbie and Amanda were luckily able to enjoy an in-person reveal, one that involved Debbie's people: Marty, Finn, Nuala and Kyna.

"Part of Brushes with Cancer is being able to have that story, because someone is going to Google this someday," Debbie said. "I hope this is a story where they can feel safe and encouraged."

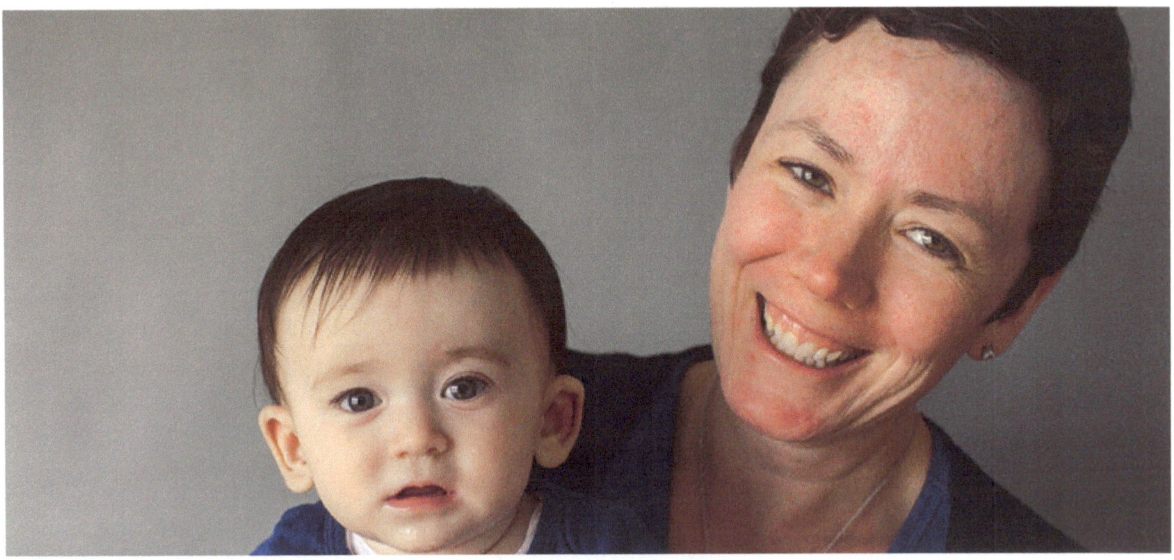

INSPIRATION DEBBIE LUBECK AND HER DAUGHTER, KYNA

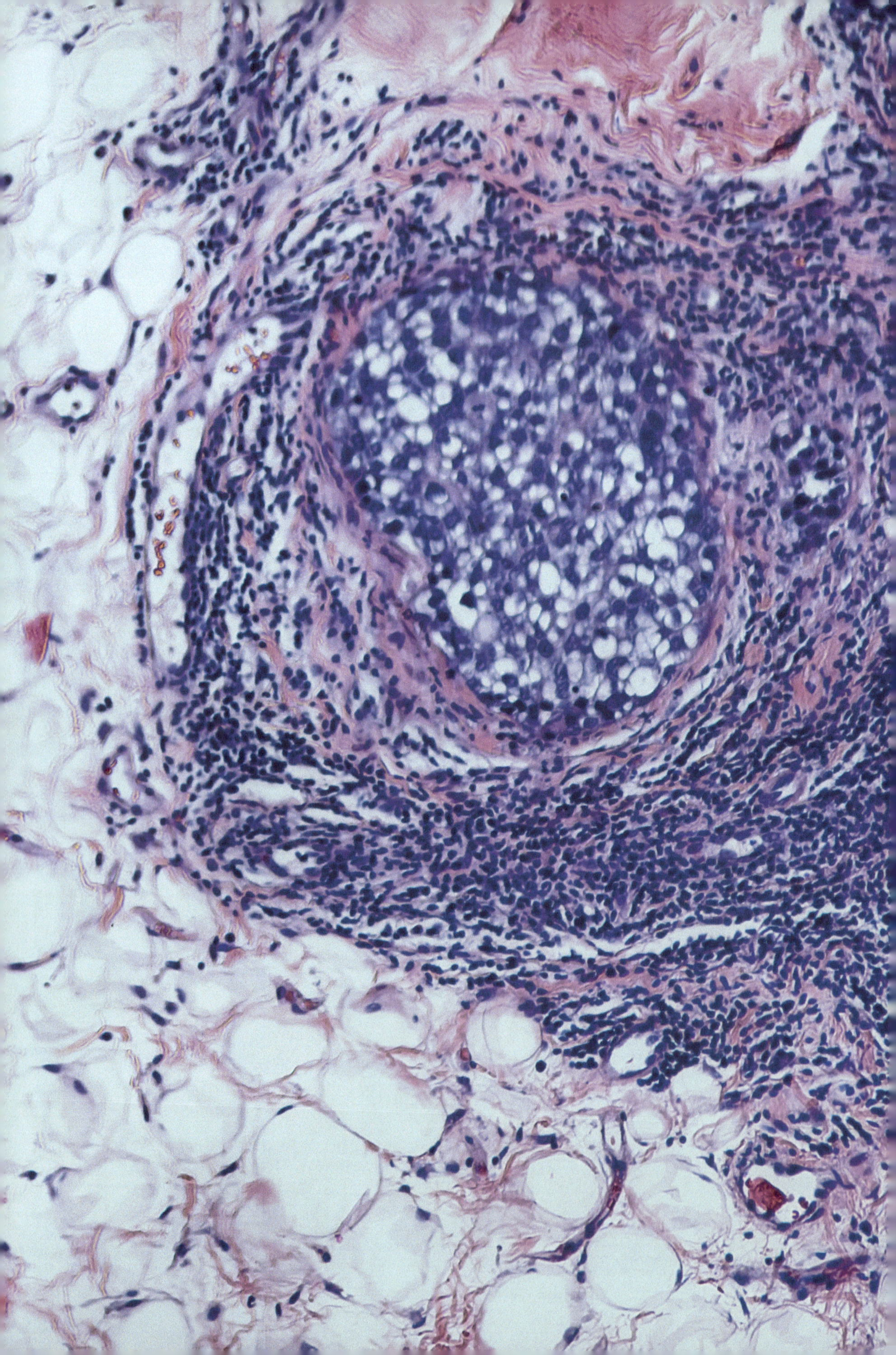

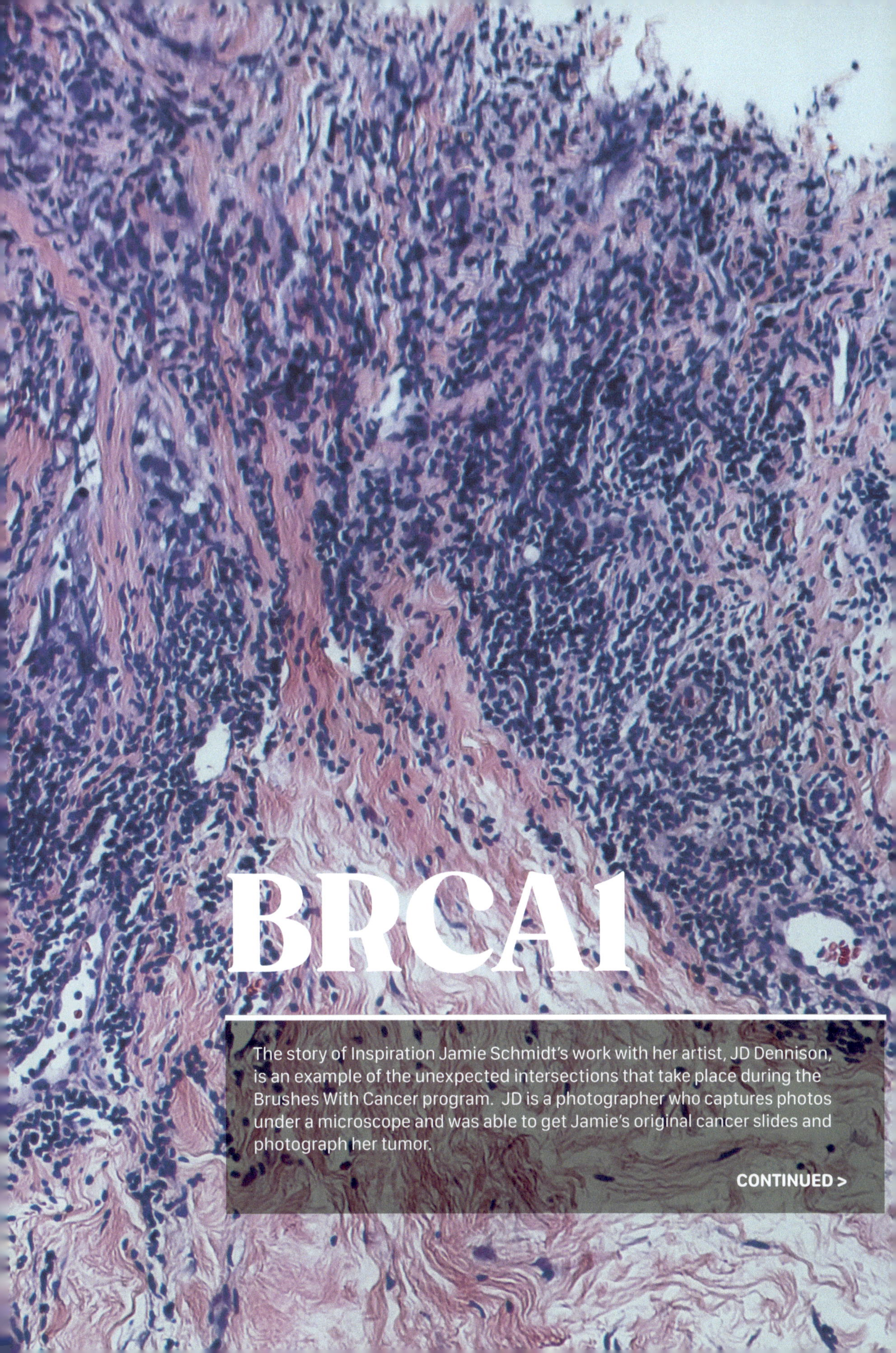

BRCA1

The story of Inspiration Jamie Schmidt's work with her artist, JD Dennison, is an example of the unexpected intersections that take place during the Brushes With Cancer program. JD is a photographer who captures photos under a microscope and was able to get Jamie's original cancer slides and photograph her tumor.

CONTINUED >

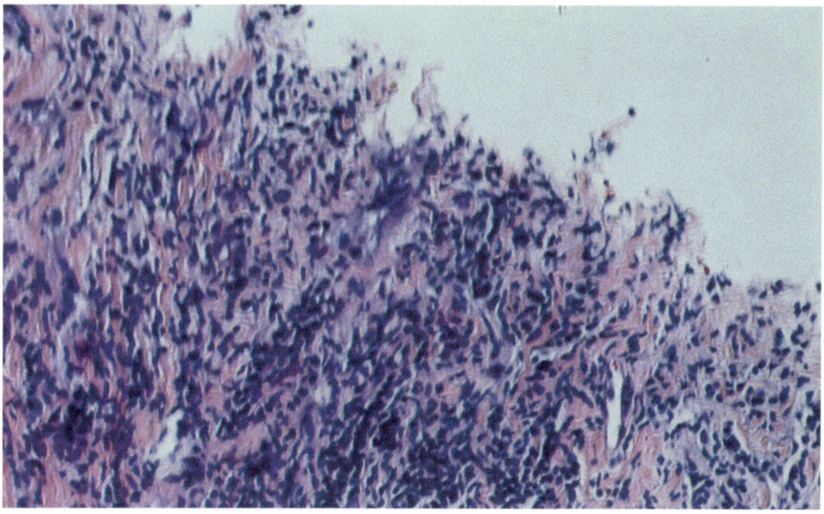

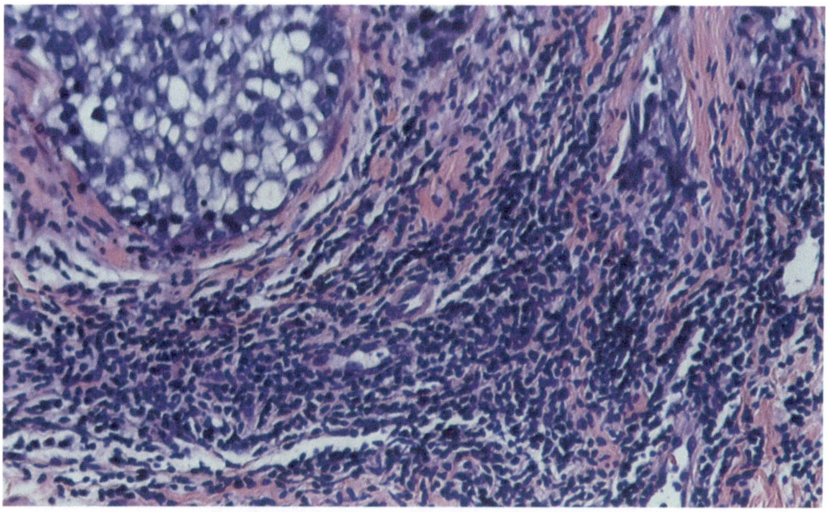

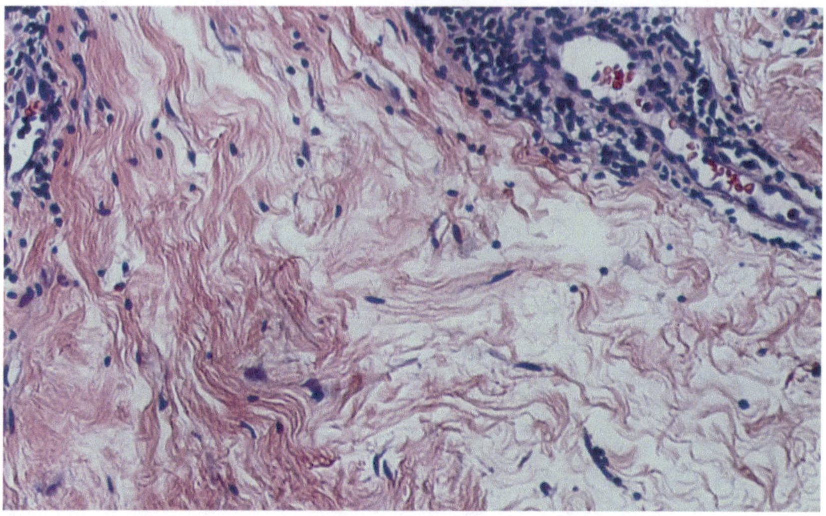

"My brush with cancer taught me to be strong and positive. Facing, fighting and living with a cancer diagnosis has made me realize that one cannot take life for granted. Life can be fragile and has the ability to change completely, especially when confronted with a health issue. However, I decided not to let my diagnosis of breast cancer and a BRCA mutation get the better of me and I took control. I keep a positive attitude, listen and follow the advice of my doctors and continue to help inspire others whenever possible. I was determined to treat and beat my cancer. Today I live with a BRCA mutation that is always in the back of my mind, but my journey has made me become a stronger person and I am so proud. 'You cannot change the wind, but you can adjust the sails.'"

—JAMIE SCHMIDT, INSPIRATION

"When Jamie and I met, we bonded instantly over discussing the science of BRCA1. My best friend's mom passed due to her BRCA gene, so it felt meaningful to focus on that. And when I discussed with our mentor my history of photographing biological tissue under a microscope, she had the great idea for Jamie to contact her hospital and request her biopsy slides! In the actual piece, I focused on the clearest example of what cancer does to your cells."

—JD DENNISON, ARTIST

"BRCA1"

Inspiration: Jamie Schmidt
Artist: JD Dennison

BWC Chicago, 2020

A Tough Nut to Crack

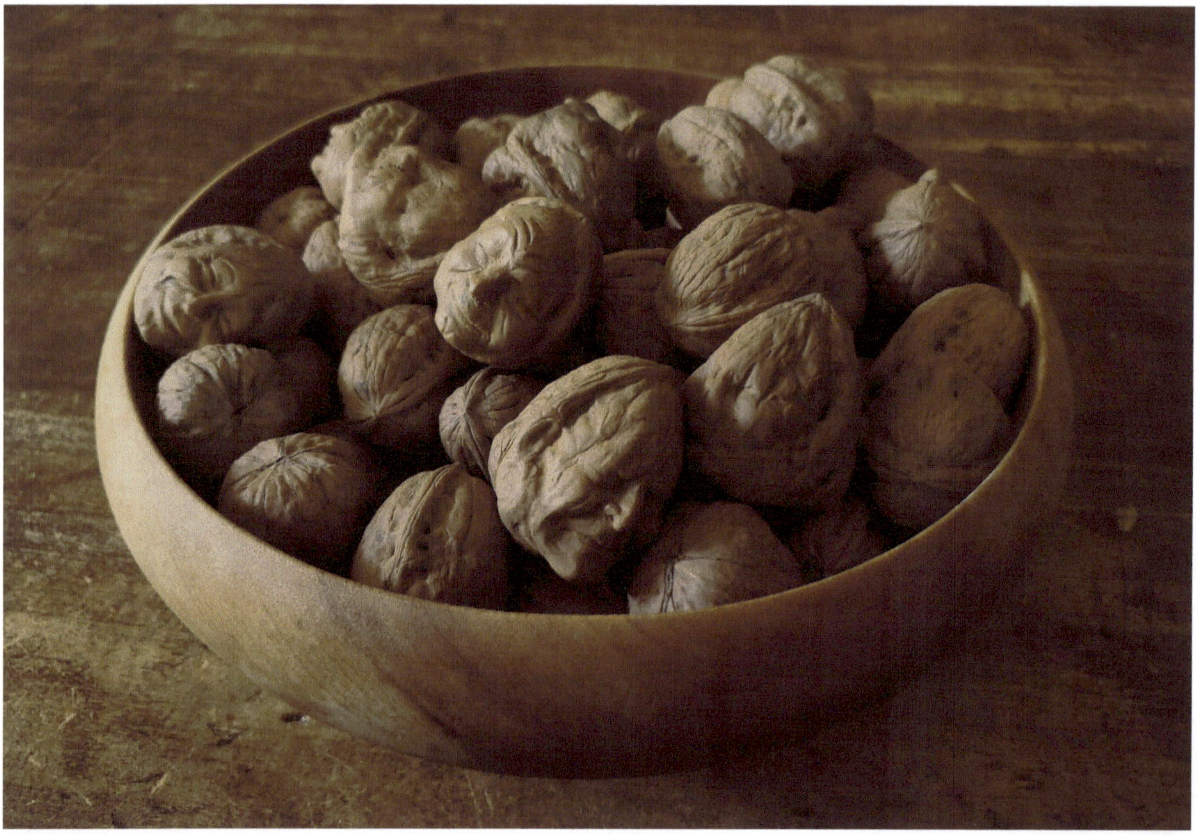

"A TOUGH NUT TO CRACK" BWC DETROIT, 2020

Carol Garrett didn't know what to expect from her Brushes with Cancer experience. One thing she did want, though, was to respect her artist's time by getting down to business right away.

> "The joy of art is coming up with something new." —KIRK RODA

It turned out Garrett's "let's do this" attitude was just one of many personality traits she shares with artist Kirk Roda. "When Kirk said 'Let's meet right away,' I said 'Yep, let's do that!' You forget and push it off. That's one of the things that resonated – if we don't do it right away, too much time passes."
Garrett knows the art process takes time and she didn't want to rush Roda, who had a big undertaking on his hands.

"I didn't know what I was going to do, what I was getting into or who I'd be working with," he said. "I wanted to jump on it right away because coming up with a unique concept takes time. I didn't want to do something that has already been done before. The joy of art is coming up with something new."

The two connected immediately and their first conversation lasted a few hours. Roda appreciated Garrett's strength and personal resolve as he listened to her story.

It was that personal resolve that inspired Roda's piece. But to really channel Garrett in his sculpture, Roda needed to listen, and listen closely. He says most of his work is based on his own intuitive trust, which is why it was important to him to really understand Garrett's story, her emotions, her personality... everything that makes her the person she is.

"I learn to trust my intuitive sense – to just go out and start," he said. "I have no idea what's going to happen, I just go and make it. After a couple hours, I stand back and get out of that area in my head and I'm surprised. For me, it's a trance-like state or extended Rorschach test. So, I wanted to gather all the info I could about Carol and her experience and let my mind go where it wanted to."

Due to their immediate connection, an idea came to Roda quickly. One challenge for Roda, however, was how to present the idea to Garrett.

"I was worried I had to make more of a sculpture she was looking for – I wasn't sure if I wanted to go that way, process-wise," Roda said. "It may be a little selfish, but I wanted her journey channeled through me. Instead of making something that would look good in her living room, I'm going to make something just by listening."

After connecting and building a deep trust between inspiration and artist, Garrett said she enjoyed her and Roda's process.

"If I could say anything to future inspirations and artists, it's: let the process flow through that discovery of what it can be," she said. "I didn't know what to expect."

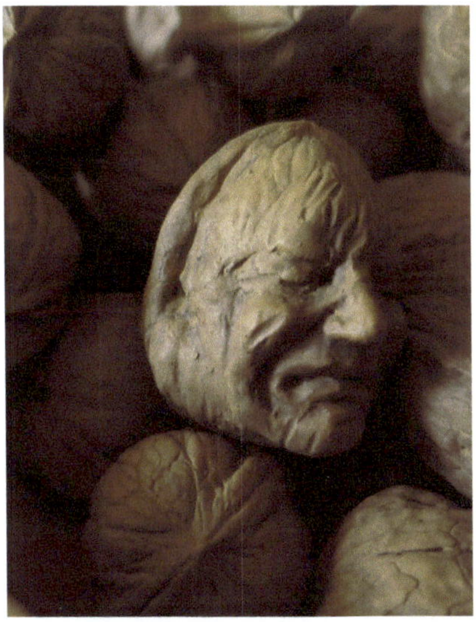

"Let the process flow through that discovery of what it can be."

—CAROL GARRETT

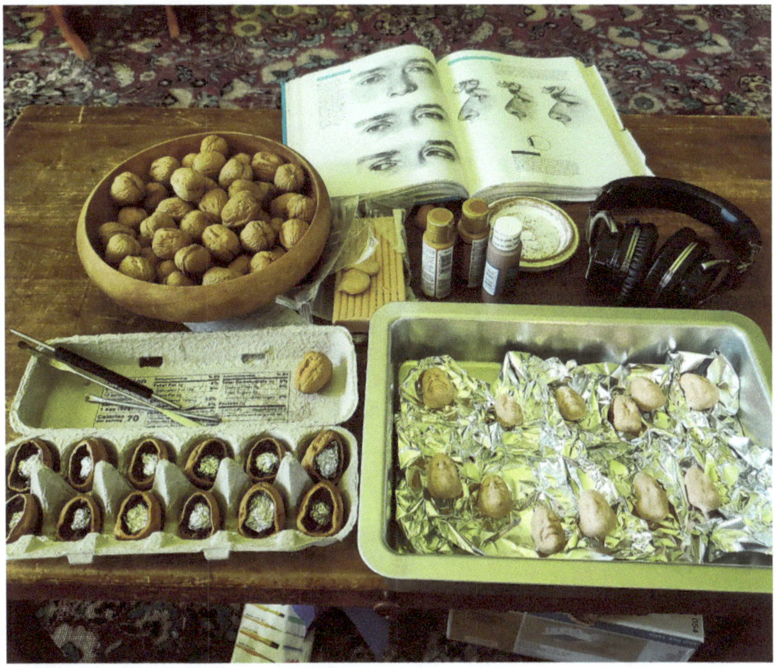

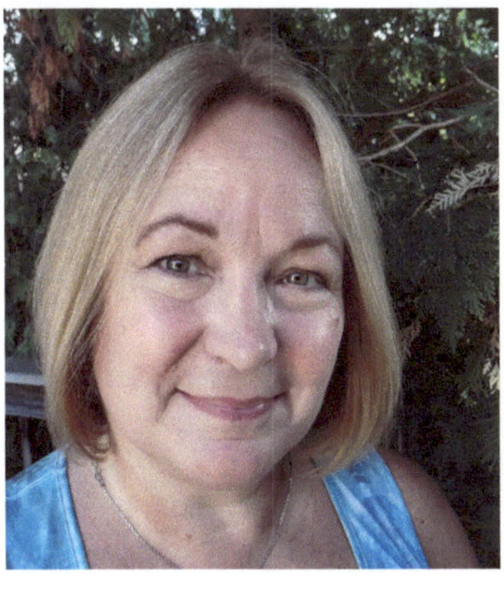

CAROL GARRETT, INSPIRATION

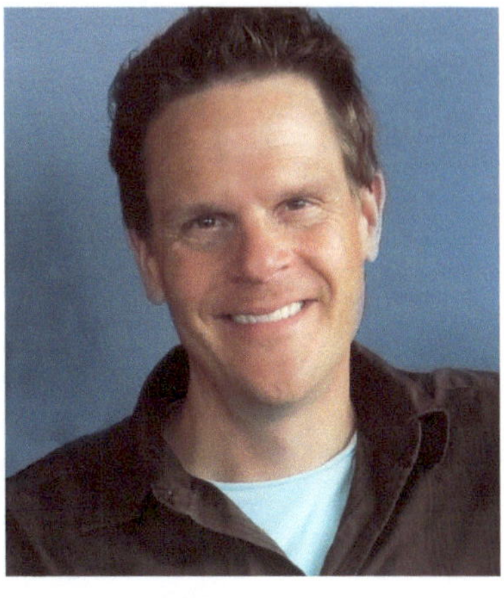

KIRK RODA, ARTIST

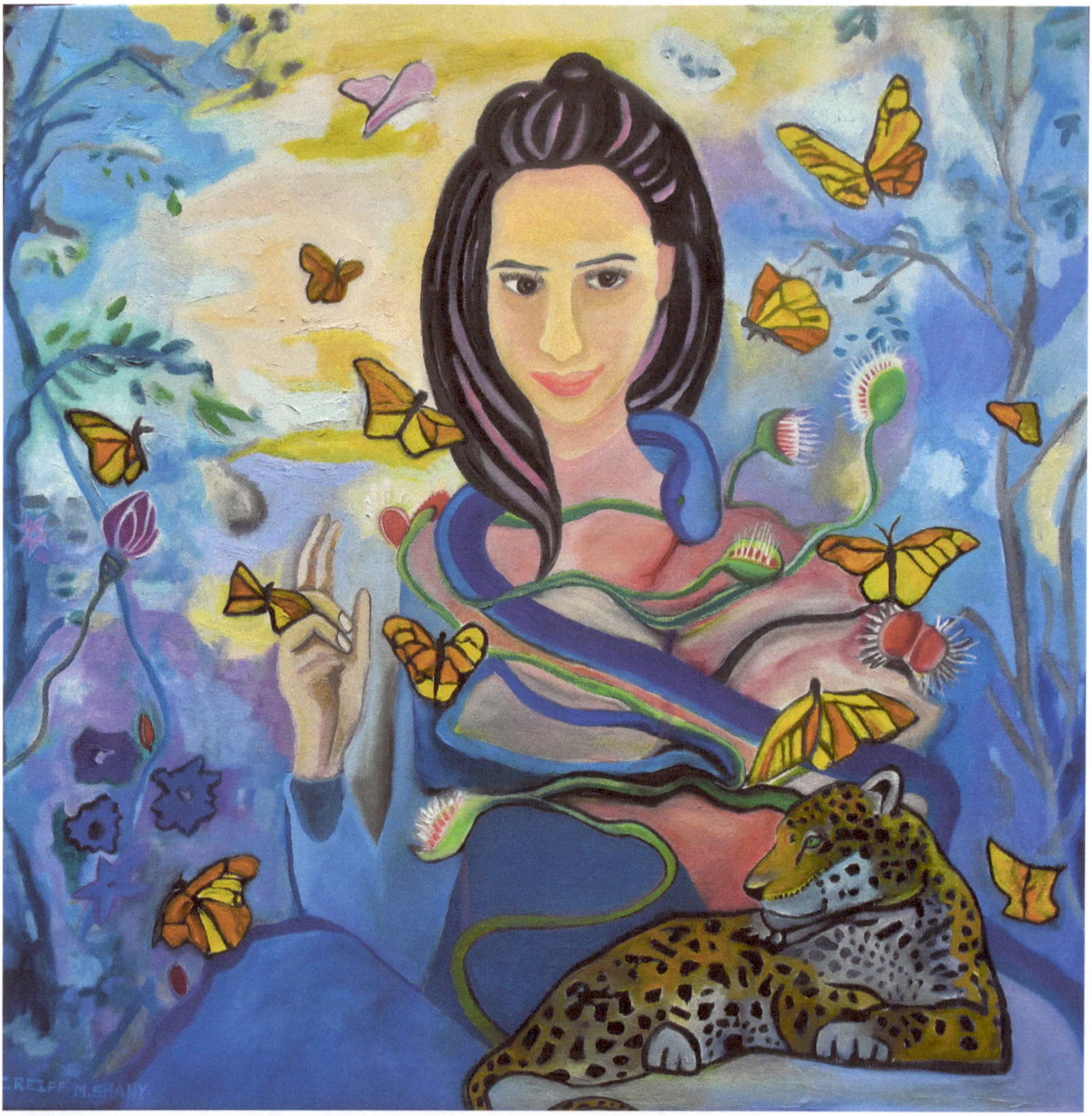

"Maya"

Inspiration: Maya Shany
Artist: Dr. Collin Reiff

BWC Tel Aviv, 2018

"I have learned a lot about myself over the past five years while living with metastatic breast cancer. Being diagnosed at the age of 26 has its unique challenges. While your close friends are defining their career paths, getting married, having kids etc. you have to find a balance between 'normal' life and hospital visits/sick days/side effects. My biggest challenge has been to understand that I have new limitations and that I can still find alternative paths and succeed. Interestingly, one can actually feel most alive during hardships and want to take full advantage of that feeling. But, in order to move forward I let myself feel the full spectrum of emotions. I turn to creativity each day as life is full of gray areas that don't follow a binary system and I always make sure to have something to look forward to. My close friend sent me an article about tolerating uncertainty and I turn to this quote often: 'reframe[ing] uncertainty as a surmountable challenge rather than as a threat'. I would never be where I am today without my family, friends, and all those that love, challenge, support, and listen. It is the people in our lives that give it meaning and help us get through the toughest situations."

—MAYA SHANY, INSPIRATION

MAY HER MEMORY BE A BLESSING

"The painting, 'Maya' attempts to capture the love, the courage, and the uncertainty experienced by Maya, during her five-year journey with breast cancer. Maya is centered in the painting with universal religious iconography, partial lotus position, halo around her head, and hand of benediction, to capture her beauty, wisdom, humility, kindness, youth and ability to unify and protect others. The venus flytraps running across Maya are carnivorous plants trying to cannibalize the healing butterflies that surround her. The snake draped across her, half wrapped around her neck, represents the subtle but lethal threat of cancer that lingers in the background of daily life. The jaguar in the foreground symbolizes Maya's strong, courageous, and resilient spirit that gracefully forges through beautiful and challenging life experiences.

Pink is woven throughout the painting, as it is the official color for breast cancer awareness. Working with Maya has been an eye-opening, humbling and inspiring experience that has fostered self-growth and a new-found friendship with an amazing person."

—DR. COLIN REIFF, ARTIST

Stories Through Song

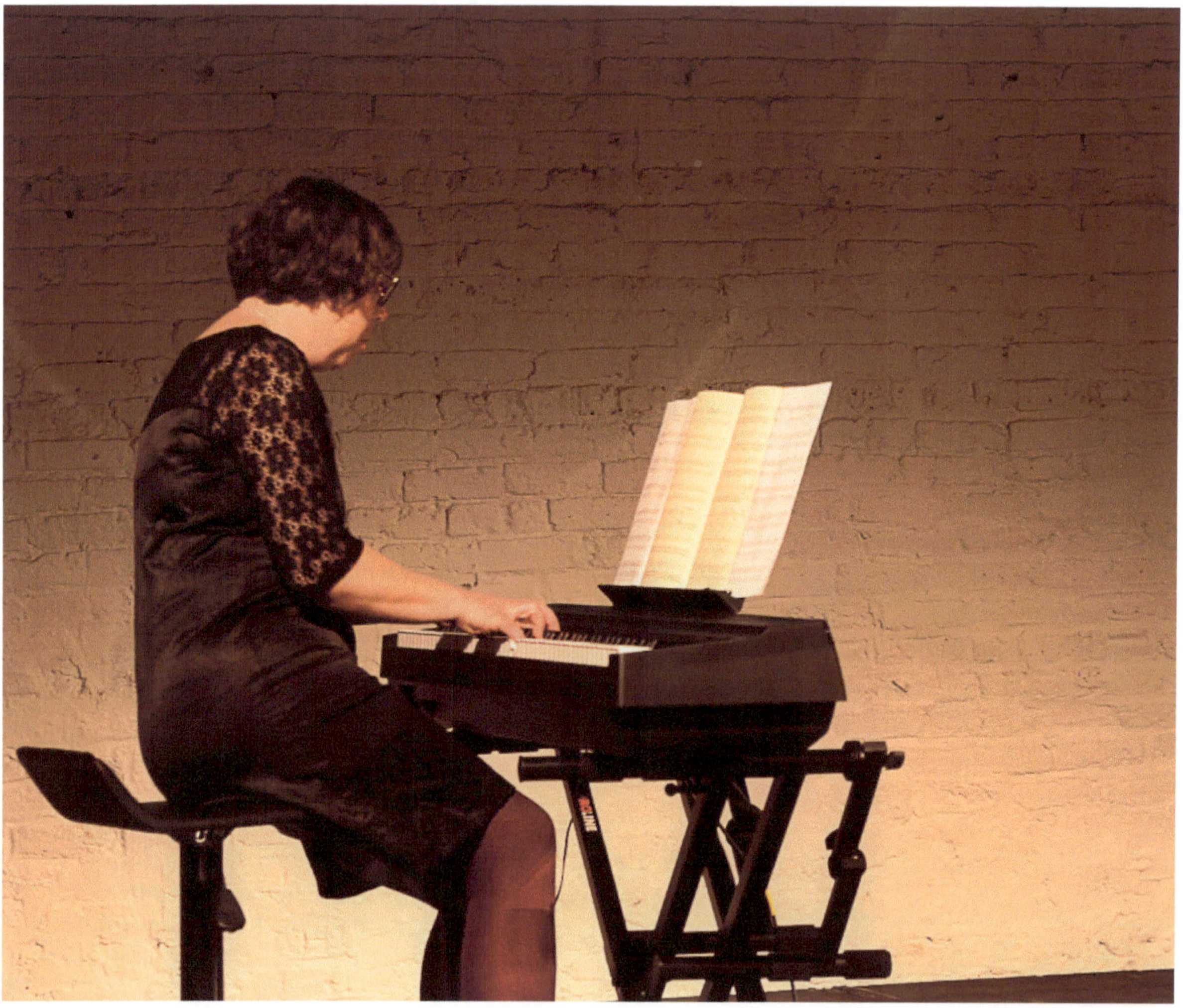

PHOTO CREDIT: DWAYNE KUAN

Inspiration: Tiffany Horstein
Artist: Jenny Conlee-Drizos

BWC Chicago, 2019

In 2011, Jenny Conlee-Drizos received information that would change her life forever: she had breast cancer. After going into remission that same year, the Decemberists multi-instrumentalist wanted to use her experience to help give back.

As she worked with different people and organizations within the cancer sphere, she was introduced to Twist Out Cancer and eventually her inspiration, Tiffany Horstein.

"A lot of cancer is like, 'Fight, fight, fight,'" Conlee-Drizos said. "With Twist Out Cancer it's, 'No, we're going to heal.' People's emotional health is super important and I love that's Twist Out Cancer's focus."

Conlee-Drizos was matched up with Horstein, a cancer survivor who got blindsided with her diagnosis as she and her husband were trying to have a child.

"A lot of things with my cancer journey have seemed serendipitous," Horstein said of connecting with Conlee-Drizos.

During treatment, Horstein and her friends saw The Decemberists perform at Taste of Chicago. A month later, she went to Portland with her husband.

"I would watch 'Portlandia' throughout treatment and I knew Jenny was Sparkle Pony on the show," Horstein said. "All those pieces connected and three and a half years later, things were coming full circle and the match was meant to be."

The two connected on the phone and spoke about their own journeys for an hour and a half.

"She was really open about sharing her experience," Horstein said. "It creates that instant connection when you hear someone else has gone through something similar. Hearing her share her story made me more comfortable sharing my story. She's so easy to talk to."

Even though the two spoke for a relatively short time, Conlee-Drizos was instantly inspired by Horstein's story. After the conversation, Conlee-Drizos wrote an outline of the major moments discussed during the call.

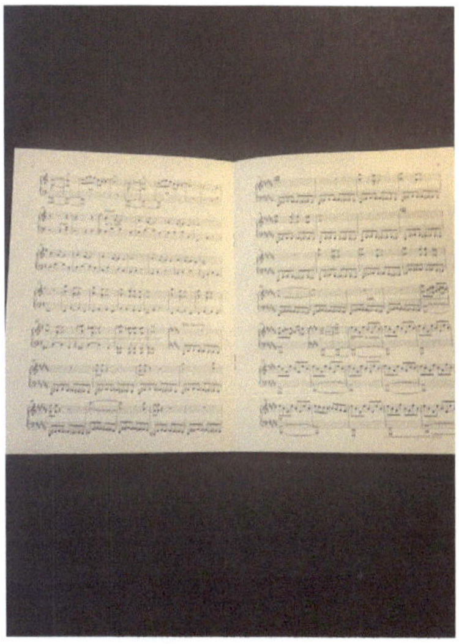
'LOOKING GLASS' SHEET MUSIC

"I sat down at the piano to find a chord progression that felt like flowing in a stream," Conlee-Drizos said of the process. The challenge was conveying Horstein's journey through instrumentals, so Conlee-Drizos explored dissonant chords and how they best illustrate that blindsided moment during diagnosis.

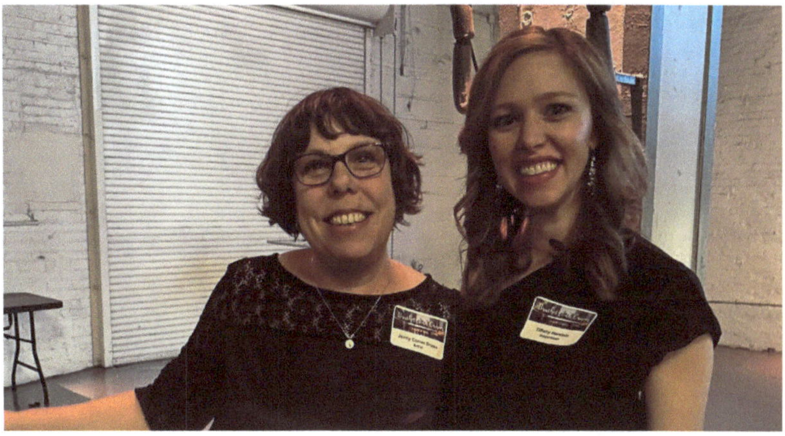
PHOTO CREDIT: DWAYNE KUAN

"My husband, Steve, said the song's end should have a dark aspect in it because life is never the same after," Conlee-Drizos said. "The feeling after the big blindsided moment and when it holds, that comes from my experience too. When you get the news and everything falls away. You realize everything in your life stops."

Being that year's Brushes with Cancer's only musical entry, Conlee-Drizos performed her piece at the 2019 event.

"I was definitely standing there choking down sobs," Horstein said. "It's so beautiful and it's not just sadness, there are so many ups and downs in the journey. For me, it was closure. It allowed me to reflect on those highs and lows. I'm still in it and not done—it's something you will always take with you—and the piece that Jenny put together displayed that. It's moving forward, it's just different."

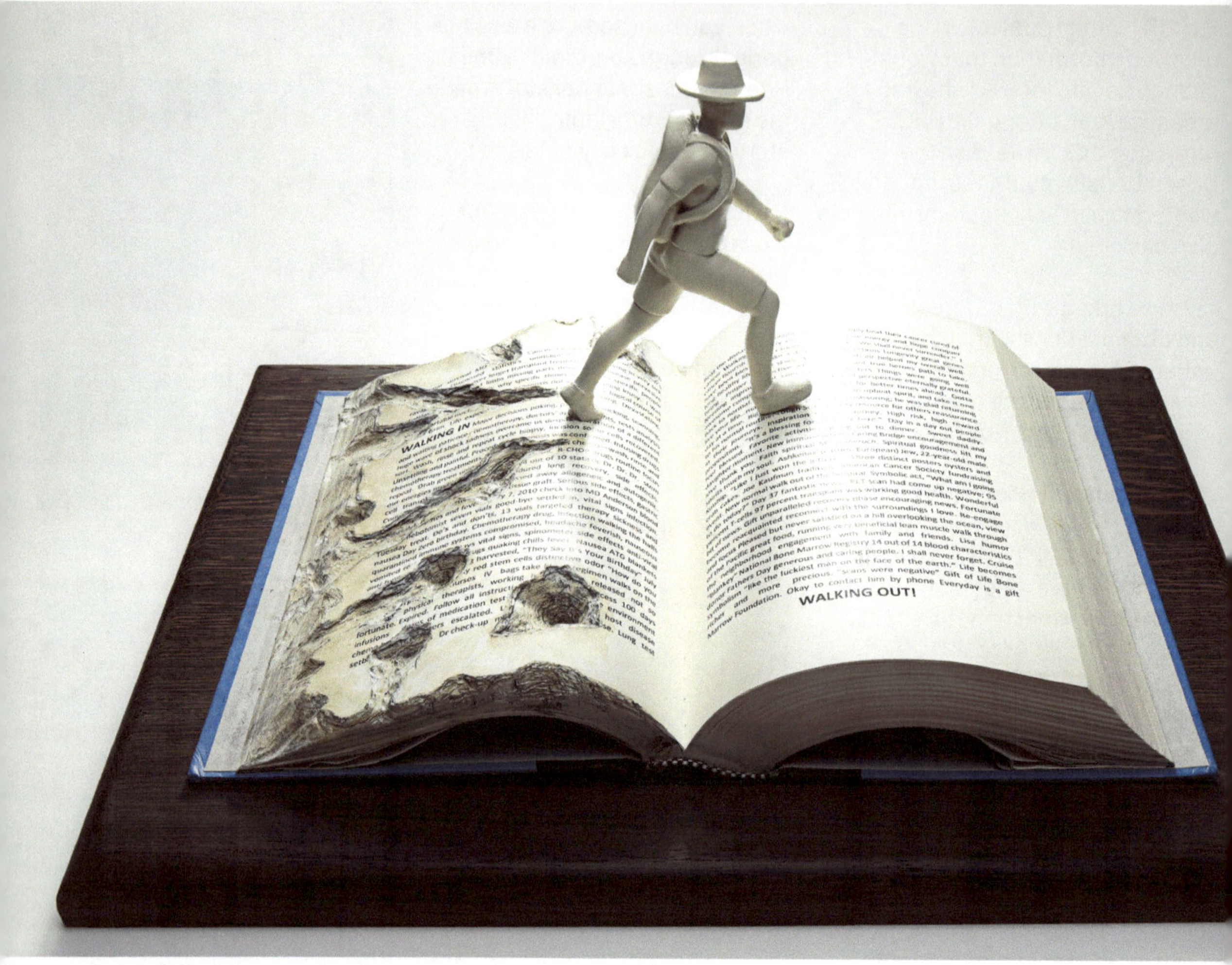

"Walking In, Walking Out"

Inspiration: Bob Kaufman
Artist: K&K Art (Bryan and Liz Kuntz)

BWC Austin, 2019

> "Stage IV Non-Hodgkin's Lymphoma in January 2009. After six months of traditional therapy, I was equally surprised to learn that the cancer had returned. Following a successful stem cell transplant in 2010, I wrote 'Replenished', as a way to provide hope and encouragement for others facing blood cancers. I believe the what-to-expect story for those considering stem cell transplants has helped others in their own battles with their disease. This was my way of giving back to the cancer community that was so supportive of me during my fight."
>
> —BOB KAUFMAN, INSPIRATION

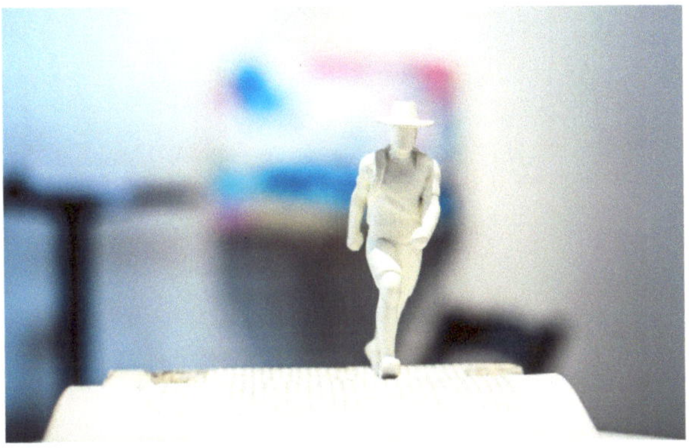

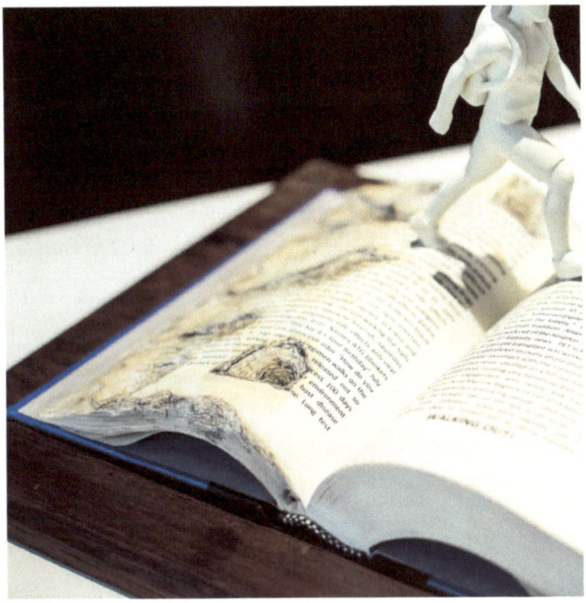

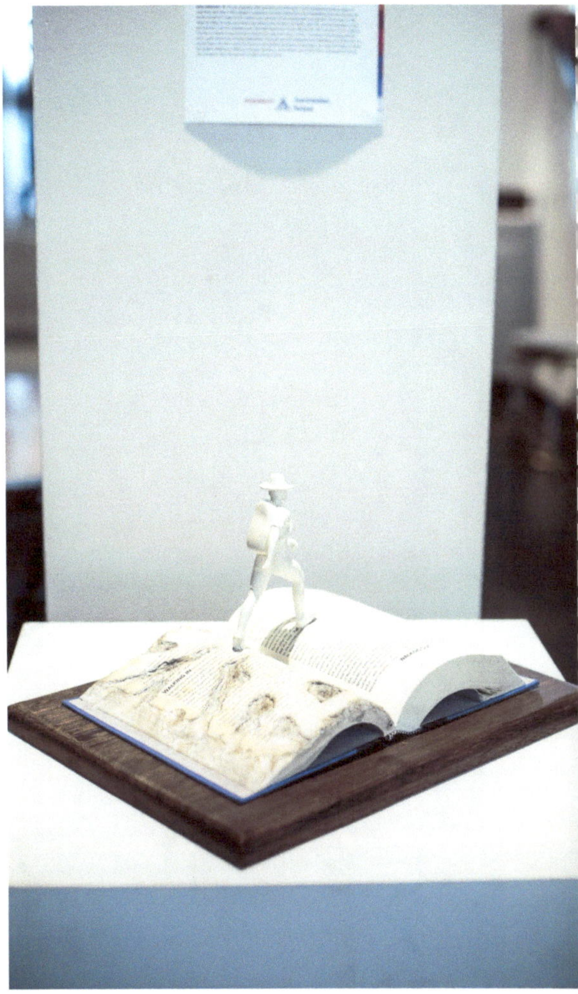

PHOTO CREDIT: LIESL DIESEL

"We met our inspiration (Bob Kaufman) one evening for a brief introduction, he told us about his experience with stage 4 Non-Hodgkin's Lymphoma. The three things that most impressed us about his story were the strong motivation to walk into the hospital and to walk out of the hospital after his treatment, that he wants to help others by telling his story, and that he now intends to live his life to the fullest extent. We used this inspiration to think and brainstorm over the following weeks. One night Bryan had a dream that was the main inspiration for the sculpture. The man is a figurative representation of Bob and his walk from cancer to cure. The words on the first page are Bob's words, taken directly from his book Replenished. These represent the unpleasant and challenging parts of his story. The second page is also Bob's words that represent the positive good days and outcomes of his story. And finally we named the sculpture 'Walking In, Walking Out' because that was a very profound part of Bob's story. It represents his strength and courage to follow through with the fight to beat his cancer."

—K&K ART (BRYAN AND LIZ KUNTZ), ARTISTS

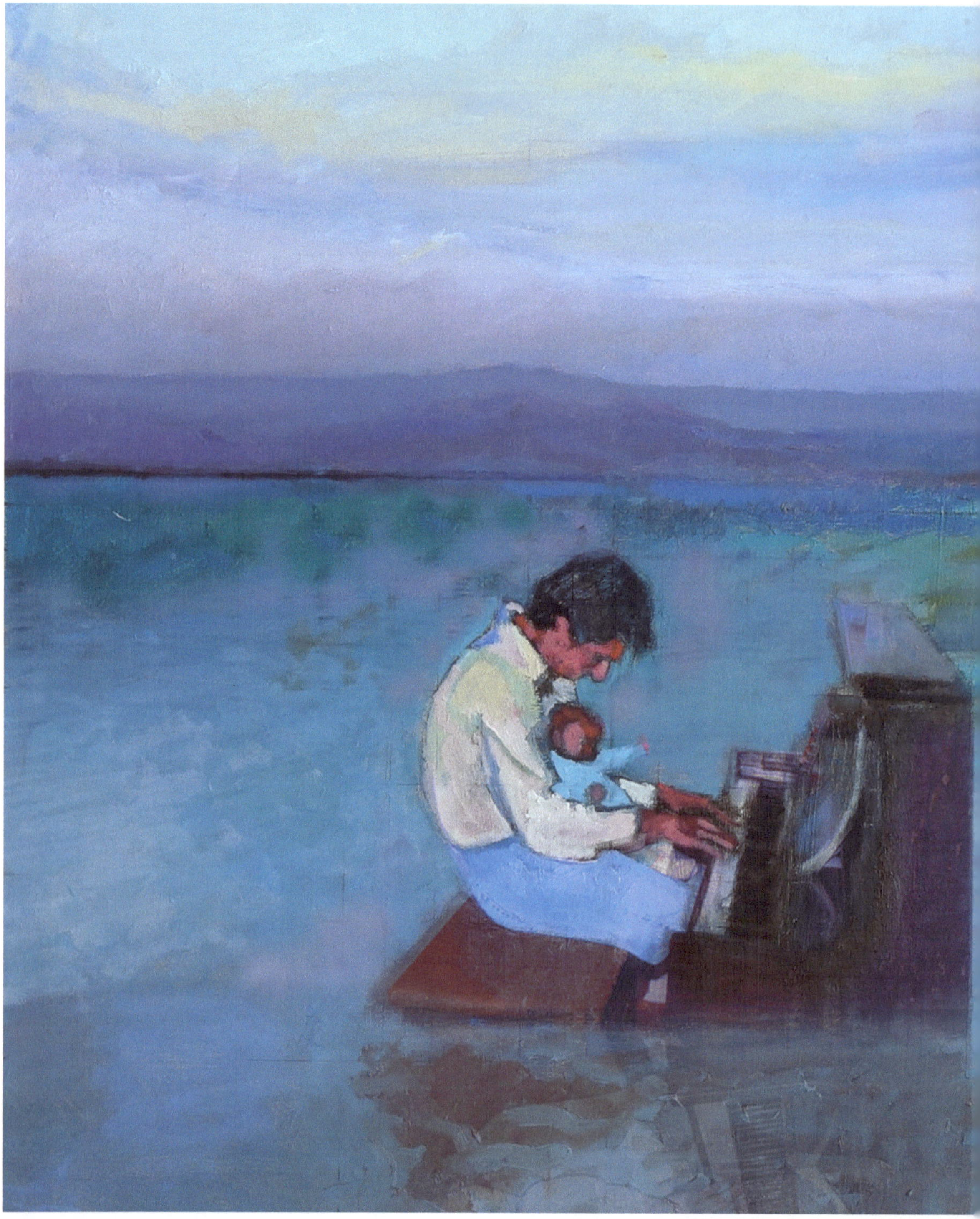

**"Things I wanted to tell you:
Mark and Aliza Ainis at The Dead Sea"**

Inspiration: Aliza Ainis
Artist: Ofer Katz

BWC Tel Aviv, 2019

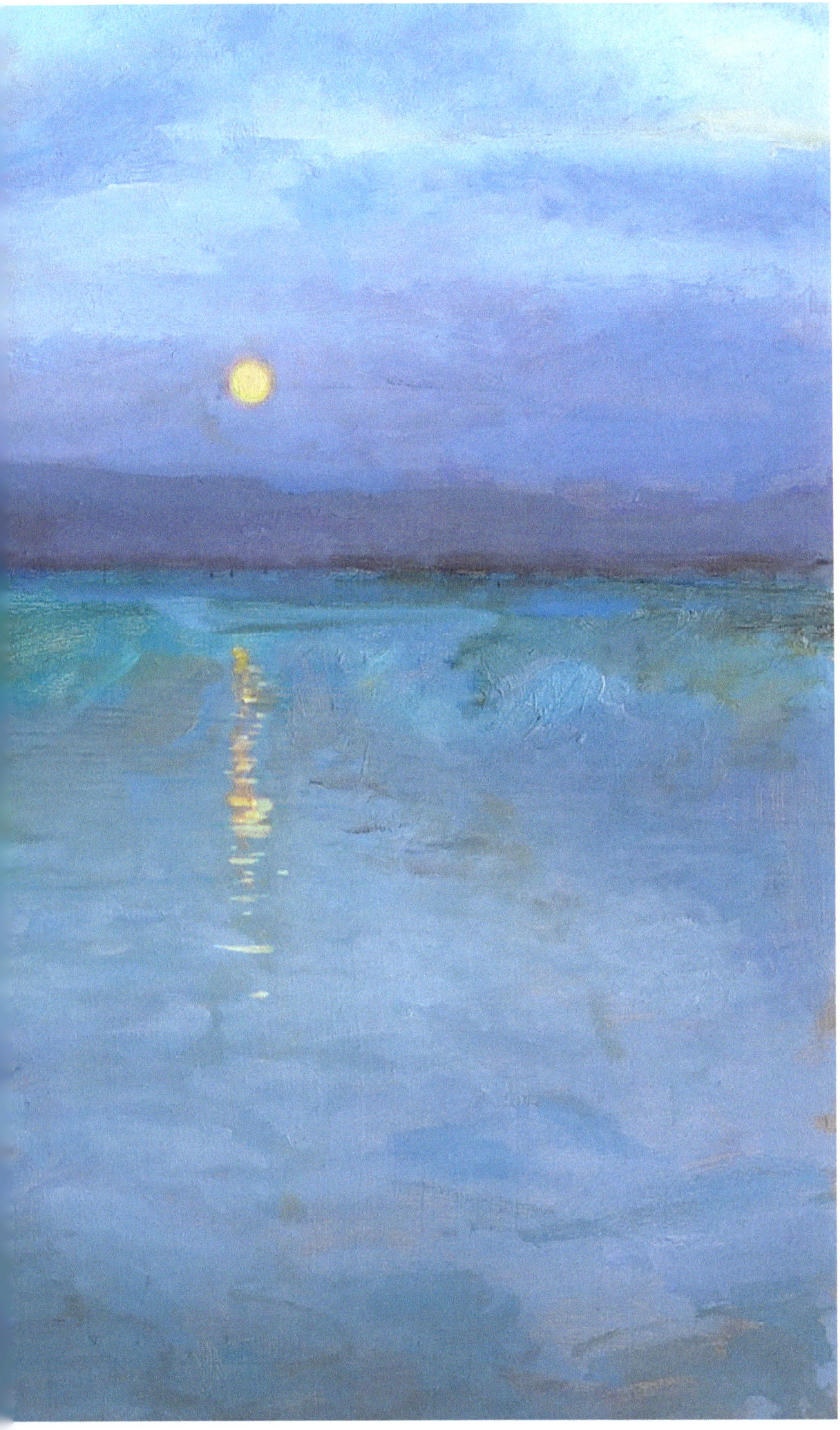

"Without the opportunity of Brushes with Cancer and the unique relationship she was able to foster through it, she may never have had the space to understand the depth through which cancer impacted her life. Her relationship with Ofer prompted her to a point of vulnerability that allowed her to invite the opportunity to heal."

The Opportunity to Heal

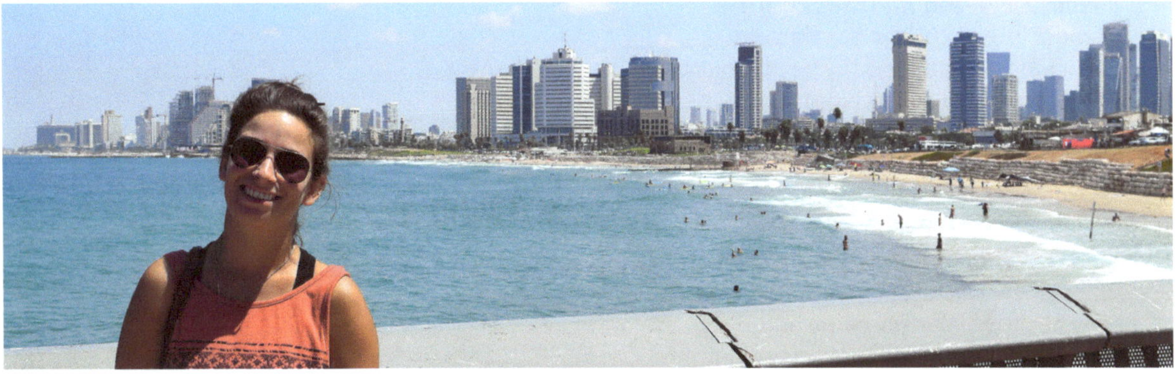

ALIZA AINIS, INSPIRATION

To Aliza Ainis and her family, creative arts were always more than just a pretty painting or a catchy song. As a musician, Aliza's father knew the power of music. Because of him, the Ainis family had creativity instilled deeply within them.

Though she may not have felt she had a natural talent for the creative arts, Aliza had something arguably even more valuable. She had an appreciation for the healing power of creativity and its ability to facilitate connection with others. Aliza said that she cannot remember exactly what prompted her to get involved with Brushes with Cancer, but it very well could have been that she holds dear the meaning of music in her family and that she was ready to heal.

Prior to Brushes with Cancer, Aliza was not fully comfortable sharing her experience as a caregiver to her father as he battled cancer. Those that were aware of her journey knew only elements of her story, but never the full scope nor the emotions that came with it. It was not until Brushes with Cancer that Aliza experienced the true meaning of connection and healing through sharing her story.

Aliza was matched with Ofer Katz, who is from Tel Aviv, Israel and relatively close to Aliza in age. Coming into the Brushes with Cancer program, Aliza describes her expectations as uncertain. Aliza's connection with Ofer was the first time she was able to articulate her experience to another person beyond a simple "bits and pieces kind of way."

Without the opportunity of Brushes with Cancer and the unique relationship she was able to foster through it, she may never have had the space to understand the depth through which cancer impacted her life. Her relationship with Ofer prompted her to a point of vulnerability that allowed her to invite the opportunity to heal.

Just like some BWC pairings, the process of creating the piece was very collaborative between Aliza and Ofer. Aliza's father was a musician, and artfully playing the piano was one of his many gifts. Throughout the process of Ofer getting to know Aliza on a personal level, she provided him with a photograph that she felt truly reflected her life and her family. That photo captured her father seated on his piano bench, gazing lovingly at his baby Aliza, as he played the piano.

After her father lost his battle with cancer around the time of her high school graduation, Aliza found herself wishing she could tell him about all that was going on in her life. Ofer describes the desire he had to "create a scene that manifests the absence of conversation, but with a presence of deep paternal love." Using the photograph as a guide, Ofer curated a piece that represents love and longing for the opportunity to share, connect, and ultimately, to heal.

"I was diagnosed with Stage 1 Breast Cancer in July 2019 at 39 years old. Cancer tested not only my health, but also my perspective on life. Normally such an optimist, I struggled to understand the purpose of this experience. It felt extremely daunting and required so much more of me than anything else I had endured. As I settled into life post-cancer and was able to reflect on what had occurred, I slowly came to the realization that going through something so challenging did, in fact, benefit me. My journey with cancer highlighted aspects of myself and my life that I was aware of, but I saw them in a renewed way and was more able to fully appreciate how special they are. There can be beauty and growth in the hardest of times."

—DANIELLE WILLIAMS, INSPIRATION

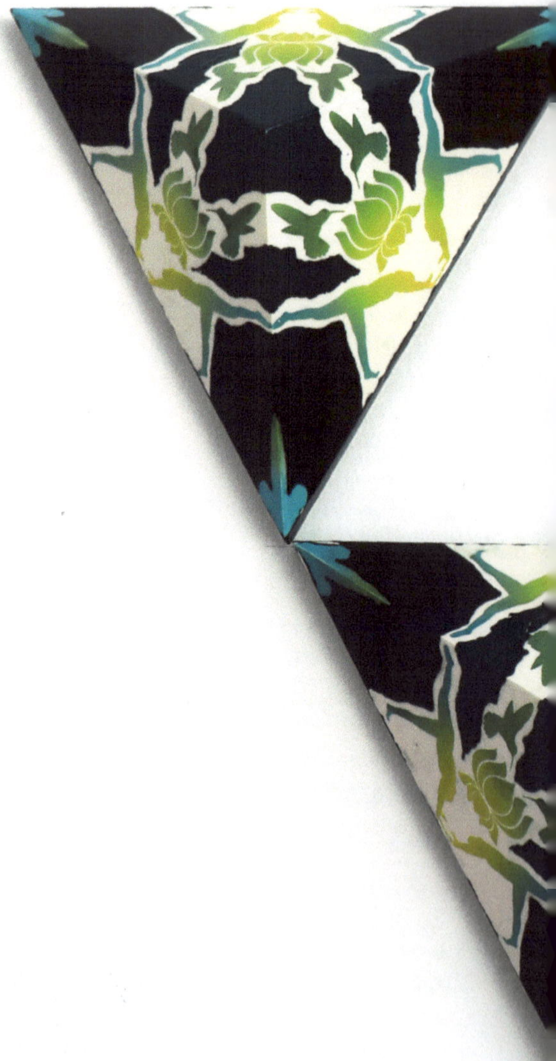

"Goddess of Feminine Strength"

Inspiration: Danielle Williams
Artist: Kara Thomas

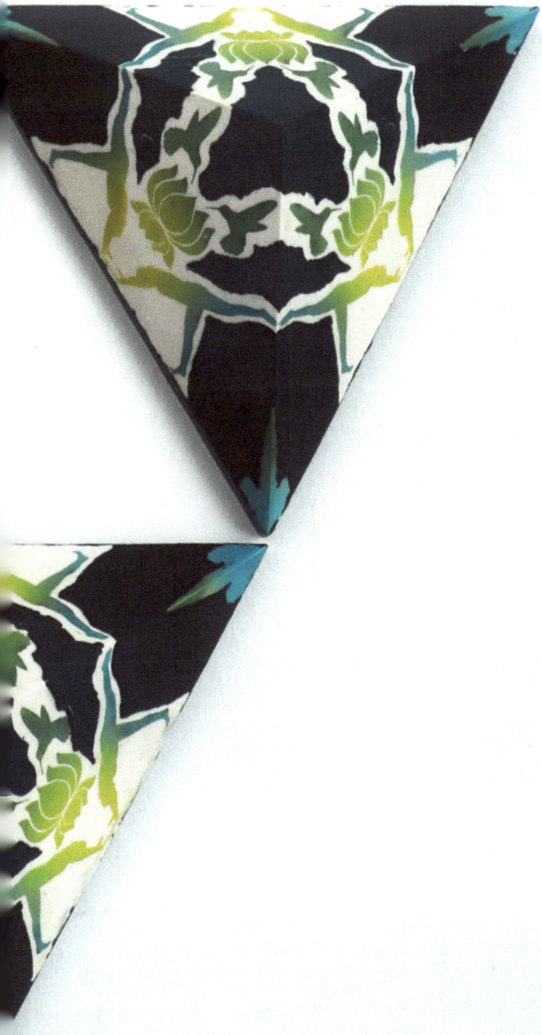

"Danielle had what she described as 'a year from hell.' Her life was changing in many ways and, on top of that, she was diagnosed with breast cancer. With not only her health on the line but feeling extra pressure with work and family matters, Danielle aimed to keep her stress level down. She practices yoga regularly and has found that in stressful situations, Ujjayi breath or 'victorious breath' used in yoga helps her through challenging times.

To represent the undeniable perseverance Danielle displayed during this time of her life, I asked her to come up with symbols that she felt represented her as a goddess. She chose the hummingbird for freedom and strength, and the lotus flower that blooms in even the darkest of waters. We took a photo of her in one legged dog, a yoga pose that she feels strong in. The image of her in this pose is also incorporated in the design. The downward pointing triangle historically represents femininity, and all of these symbols are seen dancing throughout three small triangles that make up one larger upside down triangle.

It was my pleasure working with Danielle to create this piece. Not only have I made a new friend that I have so much in common with, but am thankful for our connection that allowed me to creatively express her story. All of life's experiences are to show us who we are, and Danielle truly is a Goddess of Female Strength."

—KARA THOMAS, ARTIST

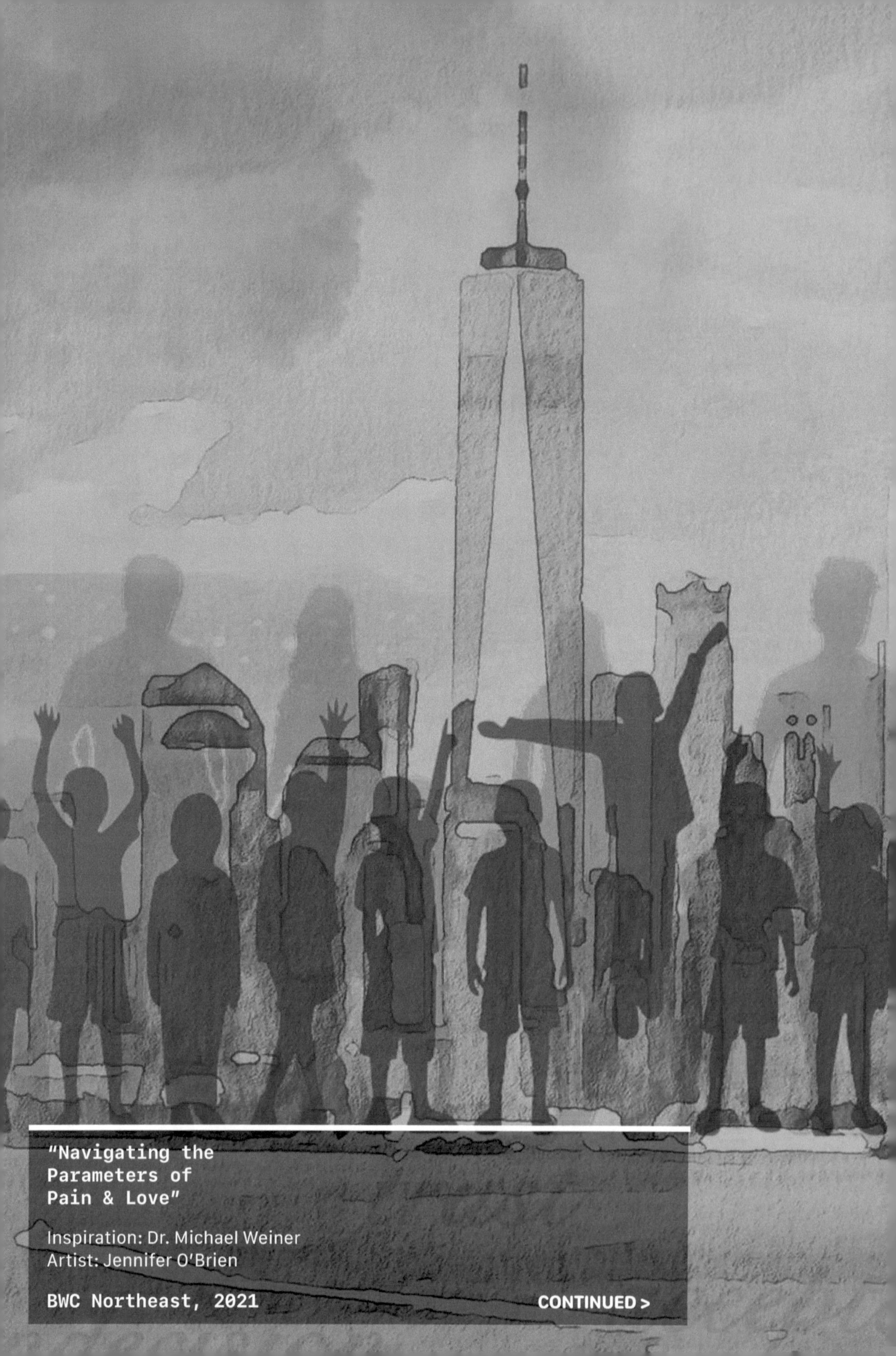

"Navigating the Parameters of Pain & Love"

Inspiration: Dr. Michael Weiner
Artist: Jennifer O'Brien

BWC Northeast, 2021

CONTINUED >

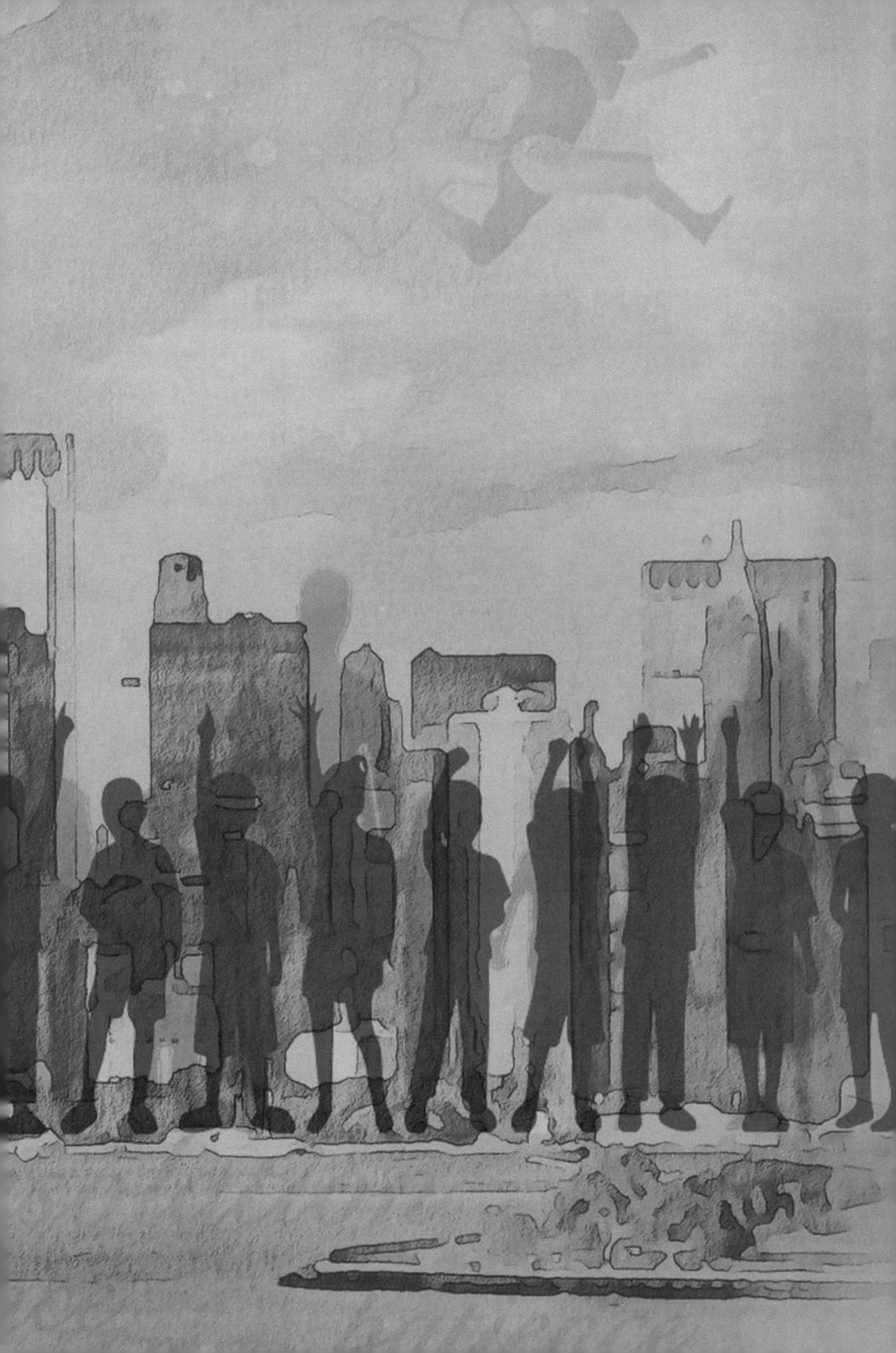

Tackling Cancer as a Father, Doctor and Survivor

Dr. Michael Weiner was no stranger to writing. Throughout his career as a pediatric oncologist, he's written scientific papers in medical literature, but adding the personal narrative aspect changed his relationship with the craft. Dr. Weiner was no stranger to writing when he published 'Living Cancer: Stories from an Oncologist, Father, and Survivor.'

"My interest in writing was stimulated by participating in these narrative medicine therapeutic sessions," he said. "This is where my career evolved. In addition to academic medical writing I now enjoy writing about my experiences as well."

While Dr. Weiner's personal relationship with cancer is touched on in the book, he makes sure the focus was on the patients who affected him the most. He carefully chose the few whose stories he wanted to share.

He recalled one patient, a teenage girl who had gone through more than many would in their lifetime. At 10, she had a heart transplant and secondary to the medication she received to prevent rejection, developed ambiguous lineage leukemia. Throughout her treatment, Dr. Weiner tried to keep her spirits up by thinking positively.

"I never take someone's hope away from them. I will never take someone's ability to think they'll be cured and be OK. Even if the odds were against survival, I felt that if one of 100 people will survive, why not you? Why not your daughter or your son?"

This young woman's prognosis, however, made it difficult to keep hope alive.

"I kept reinforcing 'I think you're going to be OK.'"

Dr. Weiner's patient, however, preferred hearing the truth.

"She said something I will always remember," he said. "Before she died, she said 'I trusted you and you let me down.' She died a day later. I felt terrible about that."

Not all stories in Living Cancer are inspirational, and that's what makes the book special. Dr. Weiner is not afraid to explore cancer's darkest moments.

A cancer survivor, caregiver and oncologist, Dr. Weiner has seen cancer in ways many have not. And through his experiences, he's learned every person is connected to cancer in some form.

"Cancer doesn't care who you are, it affects every family and it never leaves you."

Having treated cancer patients for decades, Dr. Weiner knew exactly what he needed when he received his follicular lymphoma diagnosis.

"I was not looking for a big, New York doctor. What I wanted was a partner to take me on my cancer journey and to share the experience."

He took the same approach when his daughter was diagnosed with papillary thyroid carcinoma. Knowing what it is like to live with cancer, he took his role as caregiver seriously.

"With my daughter, I decided to be her parent, not her doctor," Dr. Weiner said. "We found good people she liked and we made decisions as a team."

Throughout treatment, he put all trust in the chosen doctors, having his own career to inform which ones were best for his daughter.

It's decisions like those that make Living Cancer a unique, 360-degree view of cancer. Writing from the perspective of a doctor, father and survivor, Dr. Weiner's book is full of emotion and heart.

Dancing Alongside Tragedy

Brushes with Cancer Artist Jennifer O'Brien wants people to stop viewing cancer as a fight. The published author, artist, and healthcare administrator thinks words like "warrior" and "survivor" don't take into consideration what cancer really is. And she's right.

"It's this overused war language," she said. "It's not a fight, it's so much more – it's love, it's a sense of humor, it's negotiation with life's realities, it's acceptance, it's a lot of things. It is not a war and certainly, the people who die of cancer are not losers."

Instead, she views a cancer journey more as a dance and not a war.

"You're dancing with it, then the music slows and we have to make the dance as beautiful at the end of life as we do during life."

Throughout her life, Jennifer has had to manage this dance. Both her mother and husband, Bob, passed from cancer and at 18 years old, she lost her only sibling following an accident.

"When you have exposure to death at 18, it shapes you," Jennifer said. "It's one of the reasons Bob and I fell in love. As a hospice and palliative care physician, he understood professionally what I knew personally: that at the end of life comes death; there are no do-overs in end of life; and changed forever it is the loved ones who remain and remember."

Bob also understood what needed to be done when he was diagnosed with stage four metastatic cancer.

When Bob was diagnosed, Jennifer began an art journal.

"I wanted to document the wisdom and guidance he had been imparting to patients and families for years because we were turning it on ourselves. He was really good at what he did and helped a lot of people."

For 22 months – from diagnosis to Bob's death – Jennifer provided care to her husband.

"At first, the best for us would be a targeted therapy that would work with Bob's cancer and the worst was death," she said. "And when targeted therapies were not an option, the best ended up being quality time together."

And that's exactly what the two focused on. They lived in a large house and downsized to a condo to make things more manageable for Jennifer. They also went on a couple trips to take advantage of as much quality time as possible.

"It was wonderful we had the wherewithal to do that and Bob did that with me," she said.

"Everything we did to prepare, we would've never regretted if there was some miracle cure."

During this time, Jennifer and Bob also had candid conversations about his cancer, facing death head on. And in doing that, the dance was less overwhelming than it could've been.

"Talking about end of life when one is sick does not hasten it, and it probably makes life more comfortable," she said.

For Jennifer, death is not something you fight. It's an absolute that everyone has to accept.

"It is the one thing we all do – we don't all get married, have babies or go to college – but we all die. And if we're lucky, we love someone."

"I don't believe or say 'everything happens for a reason,' but I do believe we can learn from everything that happens. Breast cancer upended my life at 38. I had a thriving personal chef business, a husband, a teenage stepdaughter and a toddler.

By the end of 18 brutal months of treatment I was weak and tired, but I survived. My marriage and my ability to have more children did not. Though it has taken time, I have grieved all that I have lost and continue to learn the lessons only someone who has gone through certain challenges in life may ever learn. I'm following my heart and have become a birth doula, supporting and empowering others as they bring their children into the world. I have a new appreciation for and curiosity about who I am, what I want and how I want to spend my time here. For all that it has taken away, these are the gifts of cancer."

—KIRSTEN JOHNSON, INSPIRATION

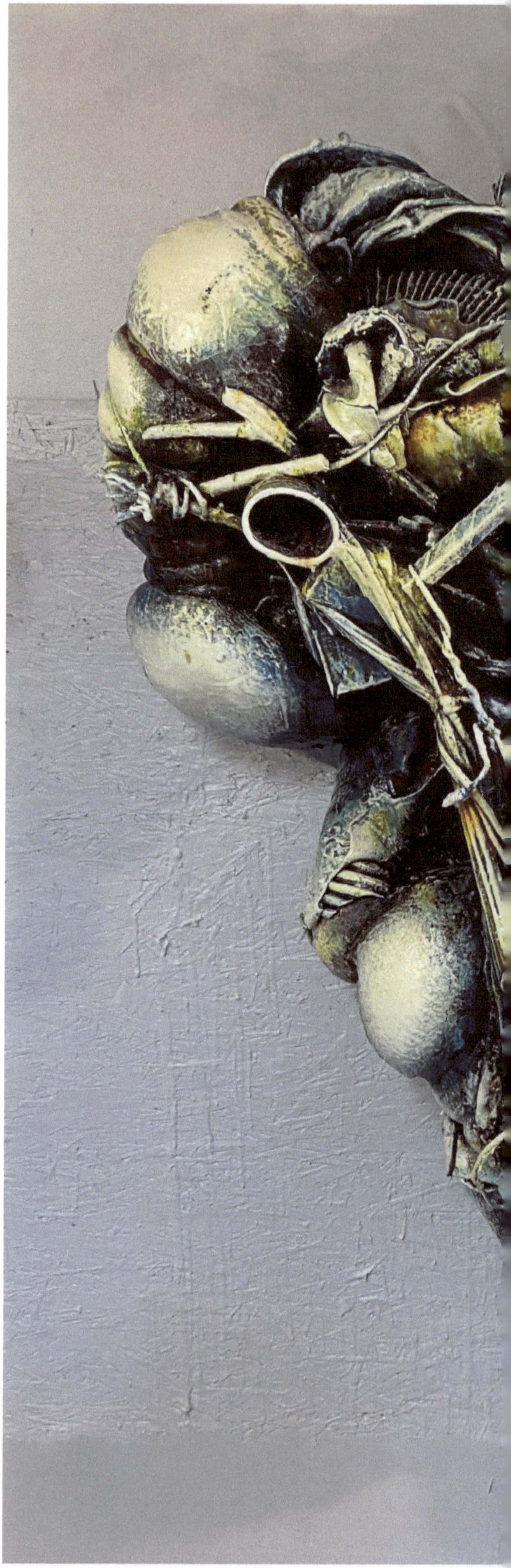

"Birth, Rebirth, and Moving Parts"

Inspiration: Kirsten Johnson
Artist: Thomas Pyrzewski

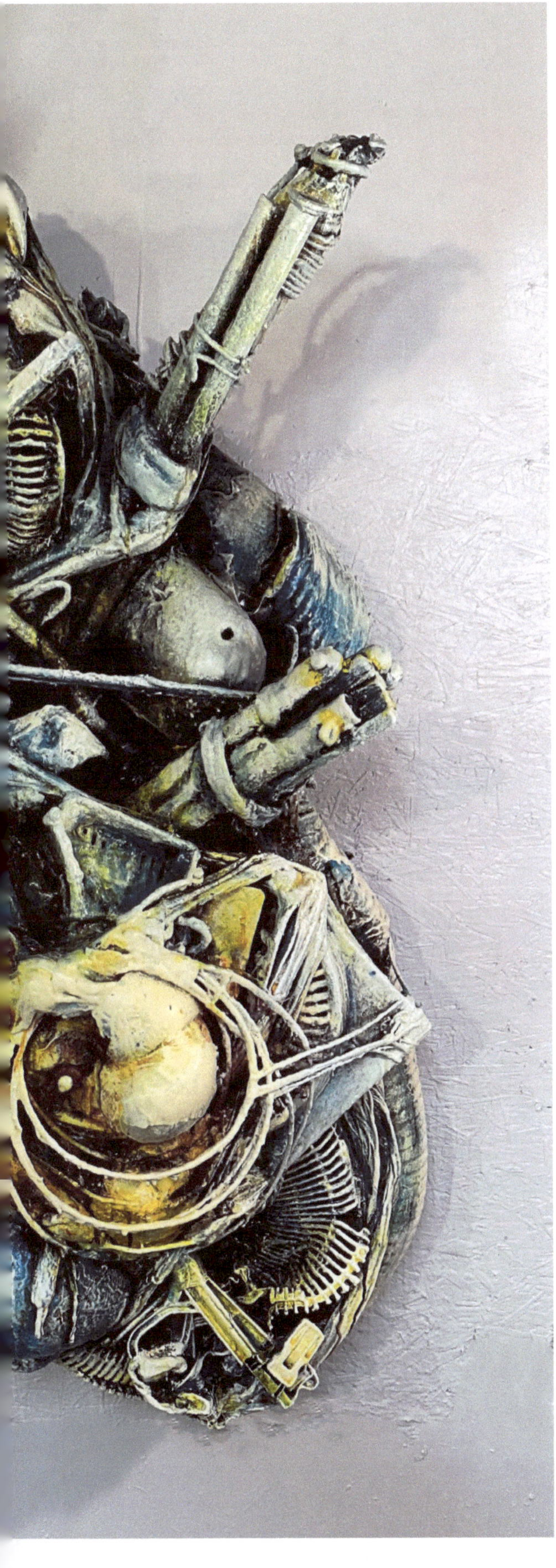

"The transition of this work from conceptual to abstract has come from discussions and implied physical circumstances. Through energy, light, and auras, our experiences were shared to heal and rejuvenate, creating a sporadic process for the construction of the sculpture. Light transcended on the form articulating a womb where a fetus emerged with warm colors, emulating hope, and new life.

I never fully understood the transitions of my work and rarely use planned sketches. This piece has created a unique opportunity to channel personal thoughts and an energy that transformed the physical.

Together, our ideas and feelings, created an understanding, an impulse to become lighter and lighter. This opportunity sparked subconscious awareness to protect and strengthen, reinforcing who we are - past, present, and future."

—THOMAS PYRZEWSKI, ARTIST

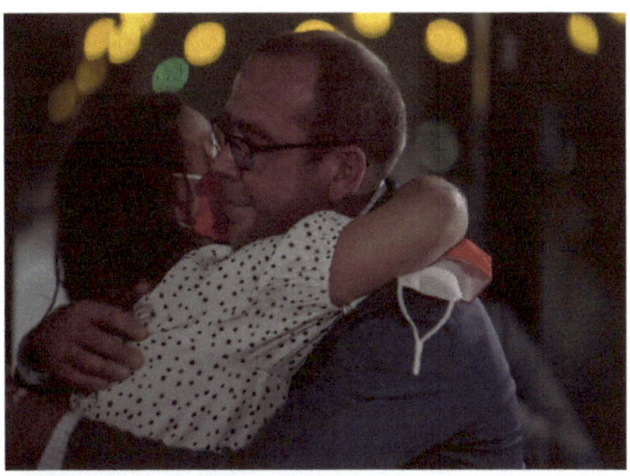

KIRSTEN AND THOMAS MEETING AT THE MIDWEST GALA (PHOTO: DARREL ELLIS)

connect

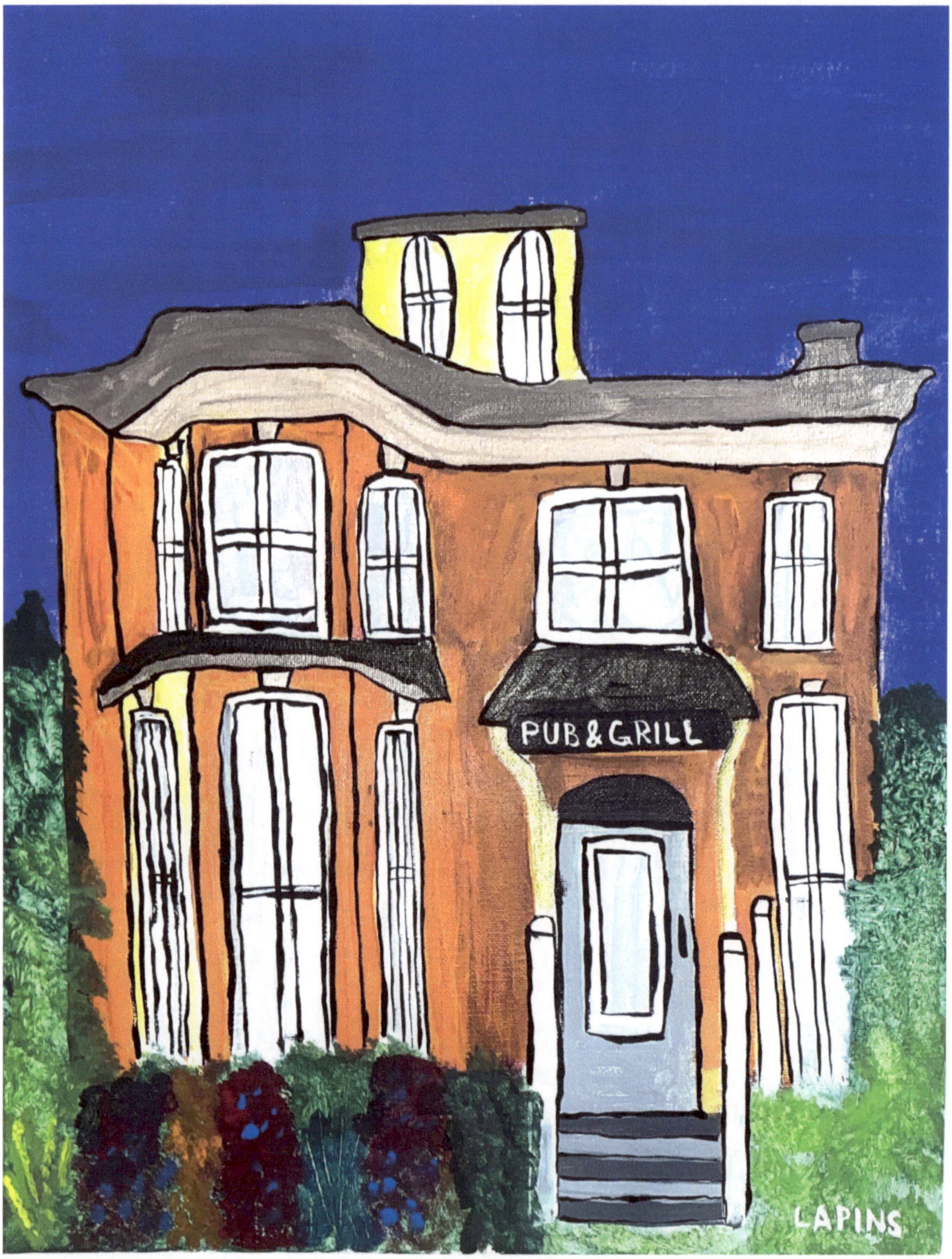

"Pub & Grill"

Inspiration: Matthew Wolniewicz
Artist: Kenny Lapins

BWC Chicago, 2020

Finding Beauty in a Downpour

To get inspiration for his Brushes with Cancer piece, Artist Kenny Lapins spent an afternoon with Inspiration Matt Wolniewicz in downtown Naperville. While there, Lapins asked Wolniewicz the places that are most important to him. Wolniewicz listed off the yoga studio, his office and Lapins stopped him.

"Kenny said, 'No. What was important while you were going through your battle?'"

Wolniewicz immediately knew and the two hopped in his car to drive to the golf course.

"To me, golfing gave me a feeling of comfort," Wolniewicz said. "Going through battle, my golfing buddies were always talking to me and when I came back, they gave me a sense of normalcy."

As the two were driving up to the course, rain immediately started pouring down. That rain quickly created a rainbow over the course and Lapins started taking pictures of the scene. He knew he had to incorporate the golf course in his piece.

"It was almost romantic," Wolniewicz said with a laugh. "Too bad I was there with Kenny."

Lapins had his sign, now he just needed to get started. Except, he couldn't.

"I start and finish most of my paintings in a couple hours," Lapins said. "I hate to leave things unfinished, and for some reason, couldn't get hooks into this one."

Although the golf course and rainbow inspired an idea, Lapins didn't have an automatic "That works!" moment when it was time to create the piece.

"This was more of a journey that he and I went through."

Lapins knew he wanted to give the piece some gravitas by exaggerating the colors and it ended up being a purple sky that jump started him.

"As soon as I put the purple sky in, I knew that was the direction to go," he said.

Lapins focused on the Pub & Grill, a dining establishment on the course where Wolniewicz goes to socialize with his golf buddies. Lapins was struck by the building's architecture and colors and as he painted, he connected to his own experiences as a cancer survivor.

"I was able to apply the things I had experienced in my journey to Matt's story and brought it to mind when I was painting."

When the painting was completed, Lapins revealed it to Wolniewicz in a text. The piece was an instant hit.

"Getting a chance to connect with Kenny and see a beautiful creation come out of a tough experience is like seeing that rainbow out of a storm," Wolniewicz said. "This has been really gratifying to me."

"Miracolo"

Inspiration: Briana Camilleri
Artist: Taylor Lazzara

BWC Chicago, 2020

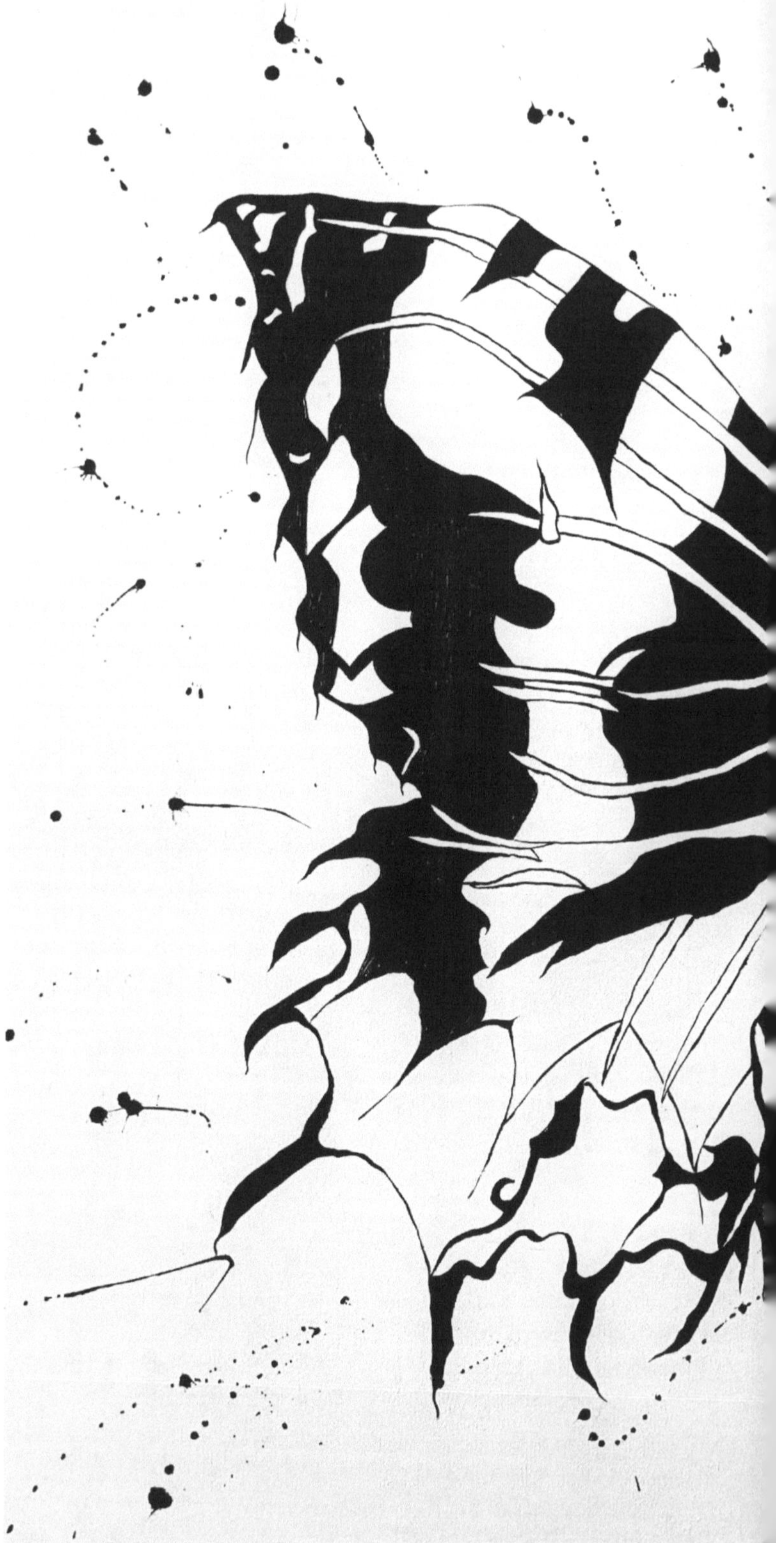

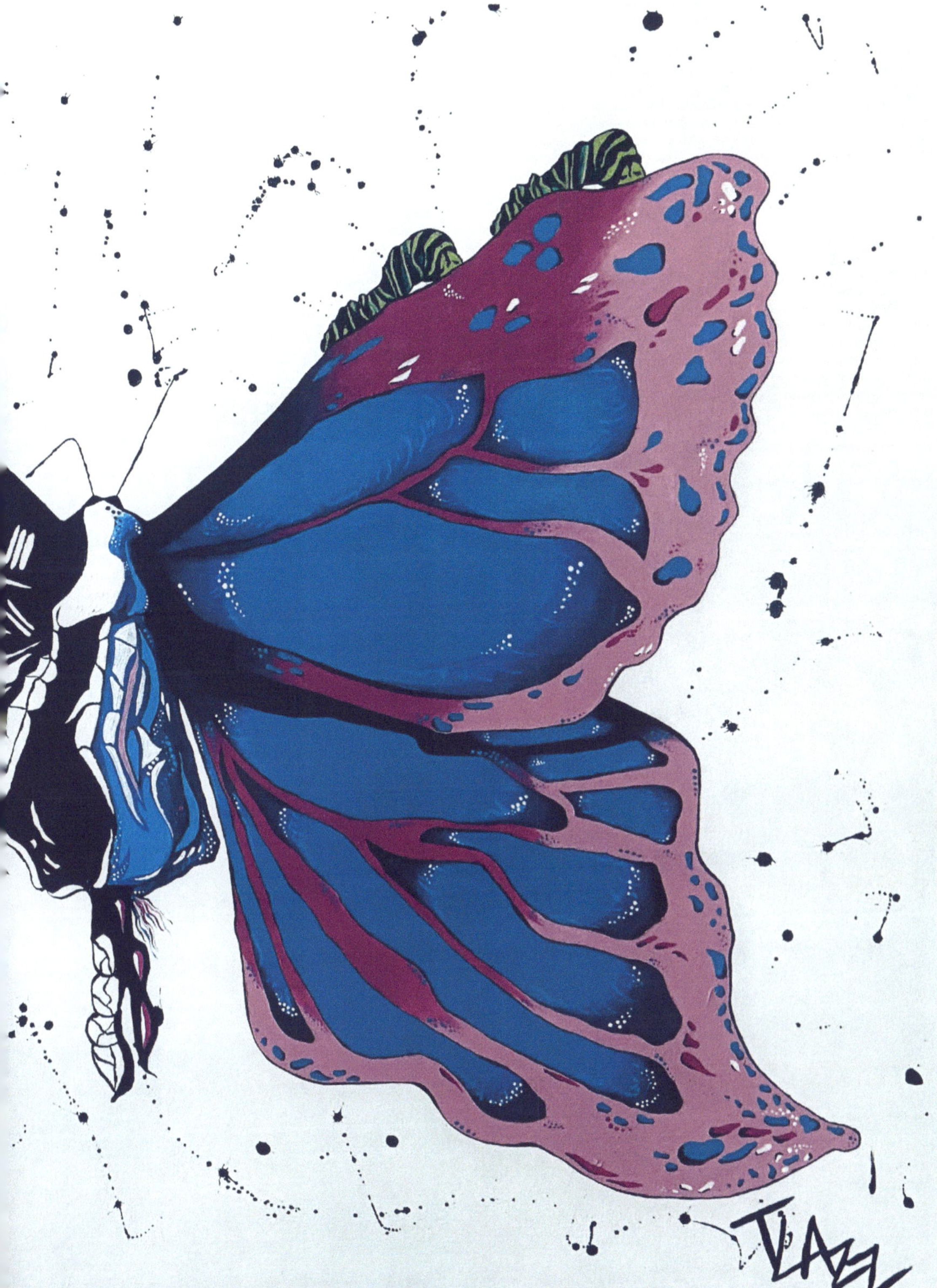

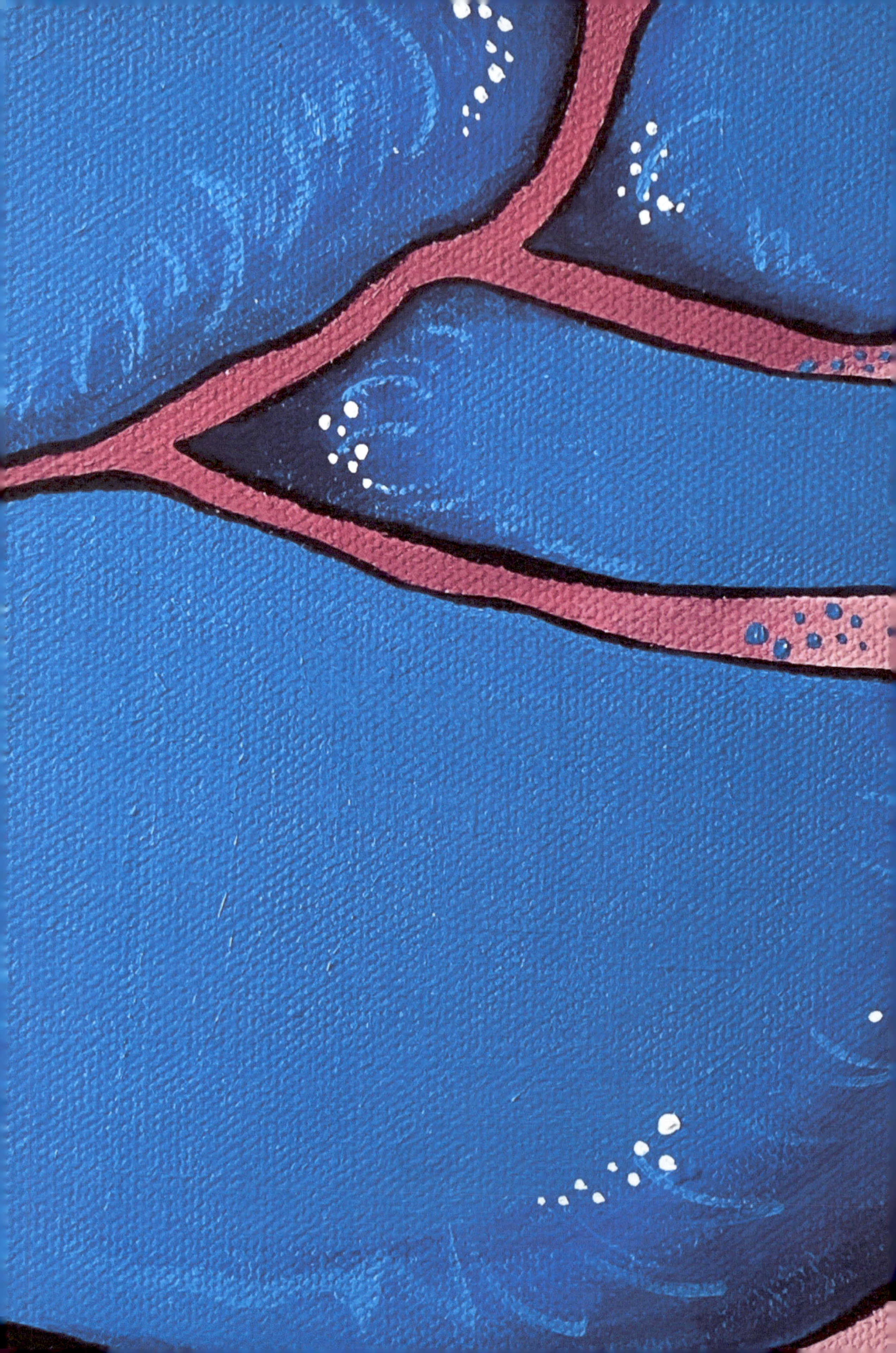

Connected Through Rebirth

When Inspiration Briana Camilleri and Artist Taylor Lazzara were paired for Brushes with Cancer Chicago 2020, they instantly connected.

"We were so excited to get to know each other that we responded to email right away," Lazzara said. "We emailed and then switched to texting – because it's more personal – then we started talking everyday, which was so neat. There are so many things that we connected on."

It didn't take long for Camilleri to feel safe putting her journey in Lazzara's hands.

"She's laid back, she listens extremely well, she's just very empathetic, understanding, funny, she can be a little crass at times, which I love. ... It's been everything I've imagined it to be and then some. I feel really lucky I got paired with Taylor."

Shortly after meeting Camilleri, Lazzara learned she was pregnant, and there was an even bigger surprise in store for both women.

A few weeks after Lazzara learned she was expecting, Camilleri received her own news: she was pregnant with twins.

"With my cancer, I was told it would be difficult to get pregnant," she said. "My husband and I didn't think it would be possible."

It was, and her due date was two weeks apart from Lazzara's. The twins were also inspiration for Lazzara, who had a few ideas sketched but threw them all out as soon as she heard about the pregnancy, which was announced in a very nonchalant way.

"I said something to Taylor like 'Do you think you can sneak in a baby?'"

"When I heard about the babies I was like 'OH MY GOD!' I knew I had to go that route," Lazzara added.

When it came to piecing together the concept, Lazzara recalled a conversation the two had where Camilleri said the thyroid gland is called the "butterfly gland" due to its shape and as the two got to know each other more, Lazzara's direction became more and more apparent.

"I wanted to be mindful of her emotions and experiences," she said. "I didn't want to focus on the heavy stuff because Bri is so optimistic. When I found out she was pregnant I decided to go this route because it's the most incredible miracle."

Lazzara used acrylic paint on a large canvas. As she worked on the piece, Lazzara envisioned it hanging in Camilleri's nursery, representing the various forms of rebirth. When the painting was revealed, it was beyond Camilleri's expectations.

"I'm just floored because it's so personal and even if it weren't, there's so much anyone could find in painting," Camilleri said. "There's rebirth in a million ways. Rebirth with cancer, rebirth with two babies. Taylor's piece has a lot of meaning to me because it's not just about the cancer."

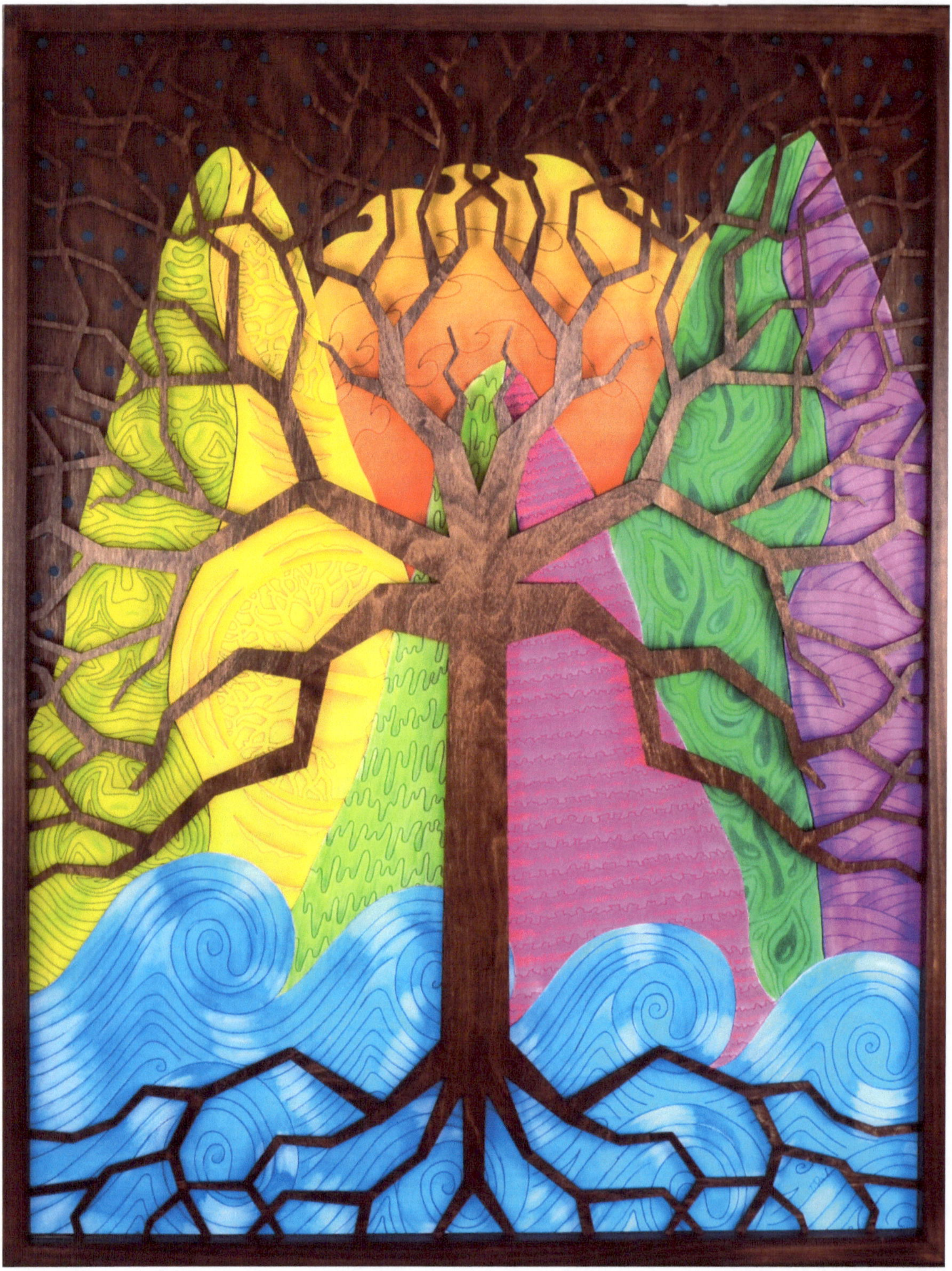

"Vacation"

Inspiration: Jonelle Binder
Artist: Tish Amparan Daniel

Where the Mountains Meet the Sea

Brushes With Cancer Inspiration, Jonelle Binder, had six tumors: five in her breast and one in her lymph node. After a double mastectomy and multiple rounds of agonizing chemotherapy, she turned to nature.

"I did a lot of energy healing. I had never discovered Reiki or energy healing before I did chemotherapy, but chemo killed me twice. It hospitalized me twice and I was very severely close to death."

Reiki is an alternative form of energy therapy that emerged in Japan in the nineteenth century. The practitioner transfers energy from their palms to the patient in order to encourage emotional and/or physical healing. Despite some skepticism of its scientific effectiveness, many people turn to Reiki as an alternative style of treatment.

"In addition to chemotherapy, I tried a natural path with supplements, prayers from church friends, and Reiki. I did a huge combination of it all. I don't know what miracle did it – but I had many miracles in my life revealed to me last year."

When Jonelle was matched with Artist Tish Daniel for the Brushes With Cancer 2020 Austin event, they had an immediate connection over nature.

"We instantly connected and shared some very vulnerable stuff on both ends. It was not all about me. There is some history in her family with cancer and she was able to open up to me about it. I was really very comfortable sharing with her right off the bat."

Shortly after meeting for the first time, Jonelle and Tish discovered their mutual respect and admiration for the Tree of Life. Tish took that information and created a beautiful laser-cut wood Tree of Life on a large, mixed media covered matte board. Flanked by large mountains and rolling waves, the multicolor shapes and designs hold various elements from Jonelle's journey with cancer. For example, the toxic green color of chemotherapy and the fiery red color of rebirth.

"She asked me what my favorite place to vacation is and I told her, 'wherever the mountains meet the sea.' And that's what she created."

Jonelle's best friend and frequent companion during hospital visits, Crystal, purchased Tish's mixed media piece, lovingly named "Vacation," during the live Brushes With Cancer auction. She lives in Honolulu, HI and Jonelle takes comfort in knowing her piece lives with her.

"Crystal and I have known each other since middle school. She is that friend that – on the day of my double mastectomy – flew in from Honolulu without telling me, and literally ran down the hallway in the hospital to hold my hand as I was being wheeled away. Then when I came out of surgery, she was right there brushing my hair, feeding my children, and loving me. She was such a huge part of this healing journey with me."

Aside from developing a remarkably close Artist/Inspiration relationship, Tish and Jonelle's friendship has since flourished beyond the event. They communicate regularly, enjoy dinner together frequently, and continue to be a part of each other's lives. Their connection is a beautiful representation of how powerful the Brushes With Cancer event is.

"Brushes With Cancer is how we connected and what she created is a part of our essence. It is so great to have acquired such a beautiful soul in my life. Our journey is melded here and I know we were supposed to meet."

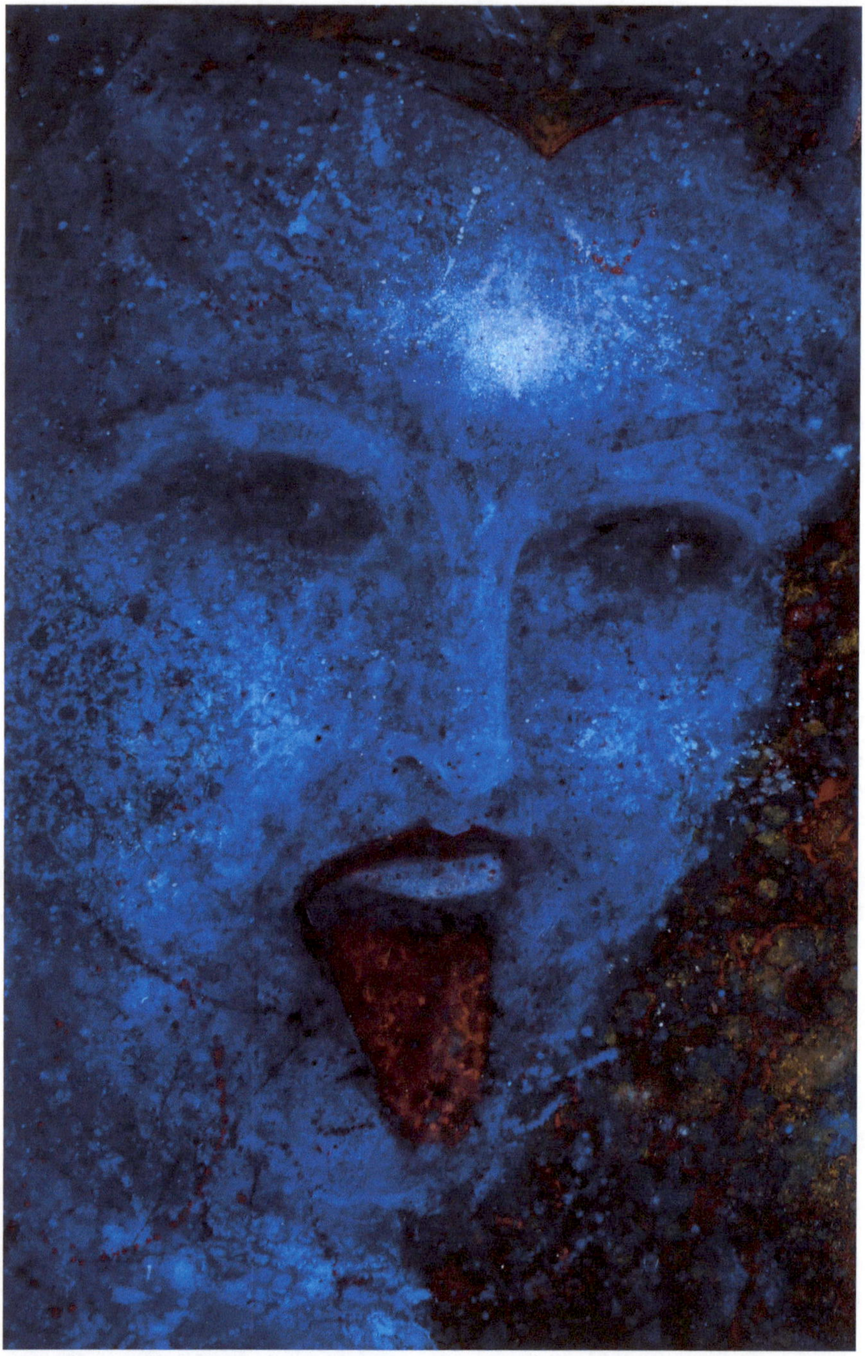

"Goddess Theresa-Kali"

Inspiration: Theresa Daly
Artist: Lauri Andreacchio

BWC Philadelphia, 2019

Feeling Seen

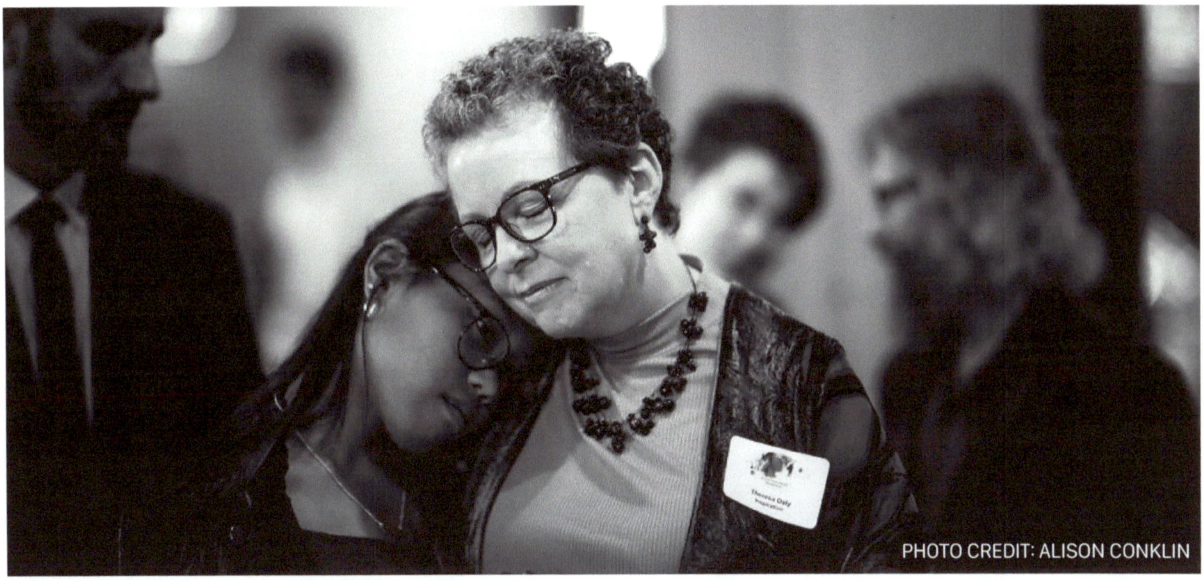

PHOTO CREDIT: ALISON CONKLIN

"The Brushes With Cancer experience allowed me to reflect on what I have been through, how I came through it, and where I am today." —THERESA DALY, INSPIRATION

Through her own Brushes With Cancer experience, Inspiration Theresa Daly was able to tell her own family about her personal journey with cancer. On the outside, she was always happy, but on the inside she was hurting. Through Brushes With Cancer, Theresa was able to bring it out and express her emotions.

Much of this was accomplished with the help of Lauri Andreacchio, who is the artist she worked with. Initially, they started communicating through text messaging. Following that, they would often get together and even do yoga together at Lauri's yoga studio.

"Being matched with Lauri has been a gift of friendship and inspiration. She is encouraging, witty and reminds me to do what I want and can do, not what is expected of me," said Theresa. "Lauri didn't look at me as someone touched by cancer, but rather as a whole person. I shared things with her that I had not yet shared with others."

Soon, their entire families were getting together to get to know each other and Lauri began creating 'Goddess Theresa-Kali,' which is the painting she made for Theresa.

"At the Brushes With Cancer gala in Philadelphia, I was so proud to see my painting hanging on the wall," she said. "People asked me about it, which allowed me to tell them about my own journey with cancer. The Brushes With Cancer experience allowed me to reflect on what I have been through, how I came through it, and where I am today."

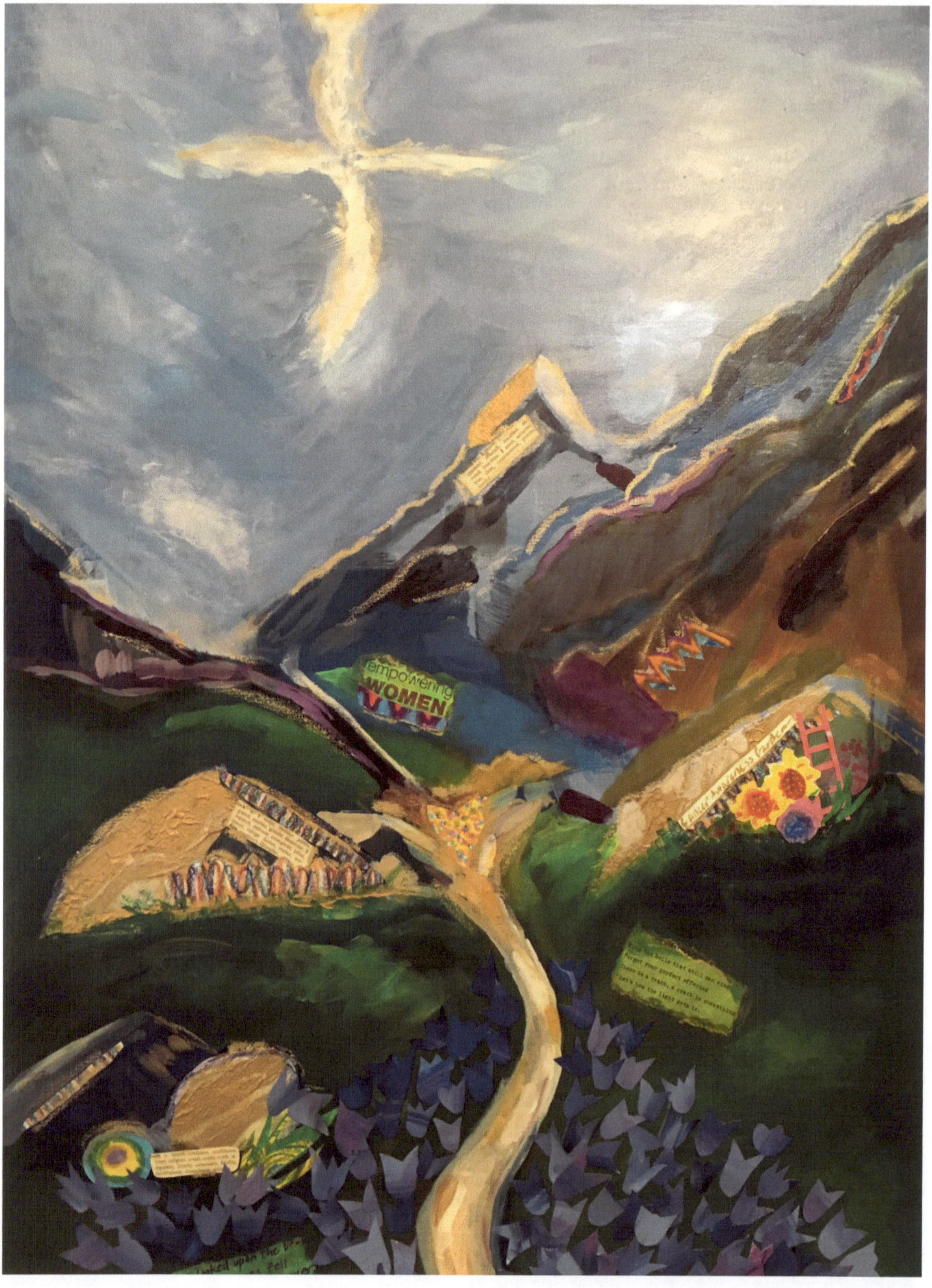

"Bluebell Mountain"

Inspiration: Karen Tabascio
Artist: Mignon Dupepe

BWC Chicago, 2019

An Inspiration's Perspective on Being an Artist

As a Licensed Clinical Professional Counselor and Registered Art Therapist, Mignon Dupepe, LCPC, ATR, has been able to see throughout her career how art can have a healing impact for both the artist and anyone that views the finished art piece.

Mignon kept hearing about Twist Out Cancer—through Jacqueline Carmody, a Twist Out Cancer staff member and Mardi Kaplan, a Board Member and Inspiration—and she knew she wanted to get involved. Mignon also had skin cancer and saw her mother pass away due to ovarian cancer.

"Through my experience doing some art projects with my mom as she battled cancer, I knew I wanted to get involved," Mignon said. "I wish this was around for my mom before she passed away."

For the 2019 Brushes With Cancer program in Chicago, she was paired with Karen Tabascio, who was diagnosed with Stage 3A breast cancer at the age of 49. They met every three-to-four weeks and Karen helped design "Bluebell Mountain," which is the painting that was made for her. The three golden mountains represent Karen, her daughter Gina, and her son, Anthony. Through several lunches they shared together, they created the collaged painted papers on the mountains.

"Through all the times we met before and after, and at the Brushes With Cancer gala, we were able to form a lasting connection. We also collaborated, and Karen would draw with some colored pencils, which I incorporated into the art piece. She had a very layered story, and I wanted to make it a layered art piece."

The practice of ringing a bell when radiation is completed was very defining and impactful

---

"I wish this was around for my mom before she passed away."

- MIGNON DUPEPE, ARTIST

---

for Karen. This powerful experience combined with her love of gardening and flowers inspired the impetus to use a bluebell theme. The bluebell flower is enchanting and is seen as whimsical and magical. Karen shares those traits of being captivating, whimsical, witty, and colorful. Karen often speaks of the idea of empowering her children, herself, and others.

This all came together at the 2019 Brushes With Cancer gala in Chicago when Karen saw the painting for the first time. Mignon and Karen hugged each other in front of the painting and discussed it in detail – Mignon pointing out parts of the painting that Karen contributed to, and Karen discussing her favorite parts of the painting. "Bluebell Mountain" is now hanging on a wall in Karen's home.

"I felt so lucky to be involved in Brushes With Cancer and am proud of working closely with Karen and telling her story," Mignon said. "May this image have the mightiest power to empower her and soothe her spirit's care."

Since that time, Mignon has become a Twistshop facilitator and has brought Twist Out Cancer's art therapy program to hundreds of people around the world. She has seen a sense of connection and community and is overjoyed in seeing Twistshop participants express their own story in a special way through their own art.

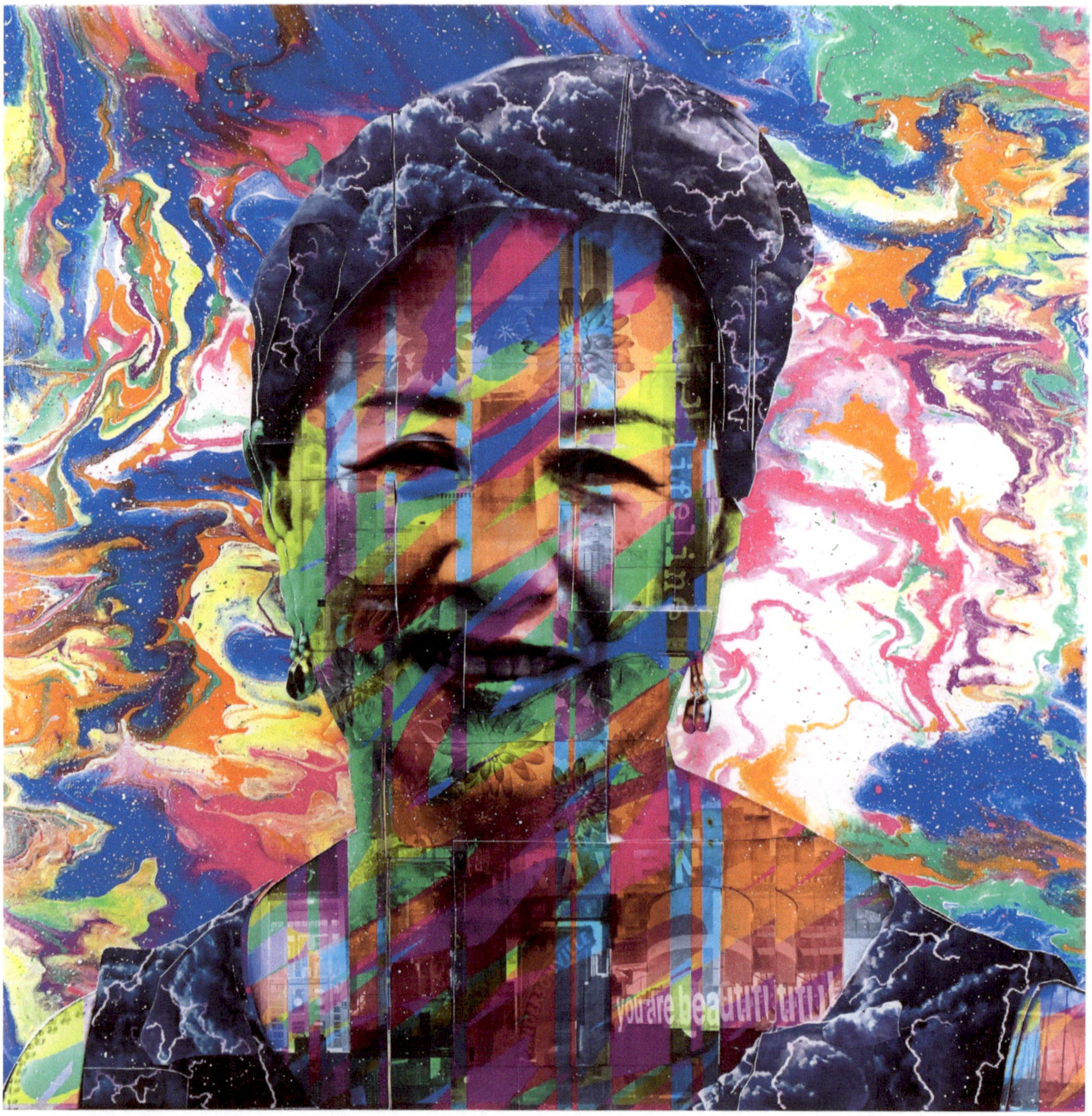

"Rainbow Lifeline"

Inspiration: Sharon Seeder
Artist: Joey Tea

BWC Chicago, 2019

An Unexpected Friendship

More than two years after taking part in the Brushes With Cancer program, "Raibow Lifeline," which is the mixed media collage that was created for Sharon Seeder, still hangs in her hallway. When she passes it, she thinks of all of her favorite places around Chicago, which are embedded in the art piece. She also thinks about the connection she was able to make with Joey Tea, who is the artist she was paired with.

Sharon was a mentor through Imerman Angels, attended a Twistshop, and then applied to be an Inspiration. She wanted to share her experience as a way to help her feel comfortable opening up. What followed was an unexpected friendship with artist Joey Tea, who is actually younger than Sharon's daughter.

The first time Sharon saw the mixed-media-collage in person was at the Brushes With Cancer gala. She was surprised that her face was part of the image and was taken aback by the amount of effort Joey put into it to capture everything that they spoke about. Joey incorporated stories and colors that Sharon mentioned into the art piece.

"Not only did Joey capture my interests in his work of art, but we became friends and met a few times after the Brushes With Cancer gala. This was an enriching experience for me, and I met a wonderful friend. I think of Joey every time I look at the marvelous work of art that he created."

Twist Out Cancer and Brushes With Cancer reminded Sharon that there are other people like her and helped her feel connected to the cancer community.

"A cancer survivor goes through feeling isolated – that feeling of 'Why Me.' Twist Out Cancer made me feel like I was part of a community of survivors."

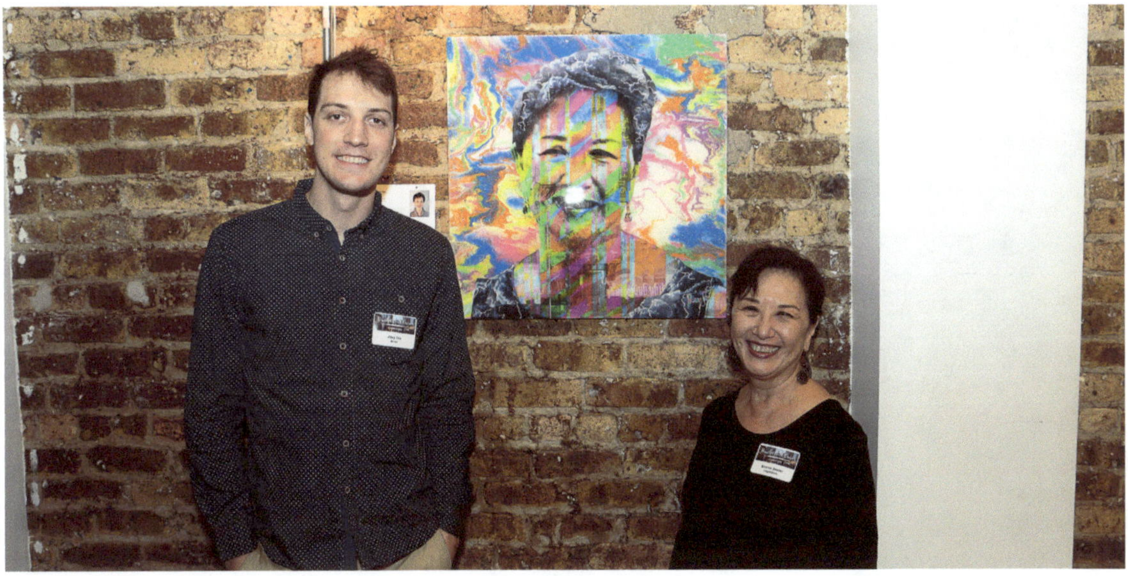

JOEY TEA AND SHARON SEEDER POSE IN FRONT OF THEIR COLLABORATION PHOTO CREDIT: DWAYNE KUAN

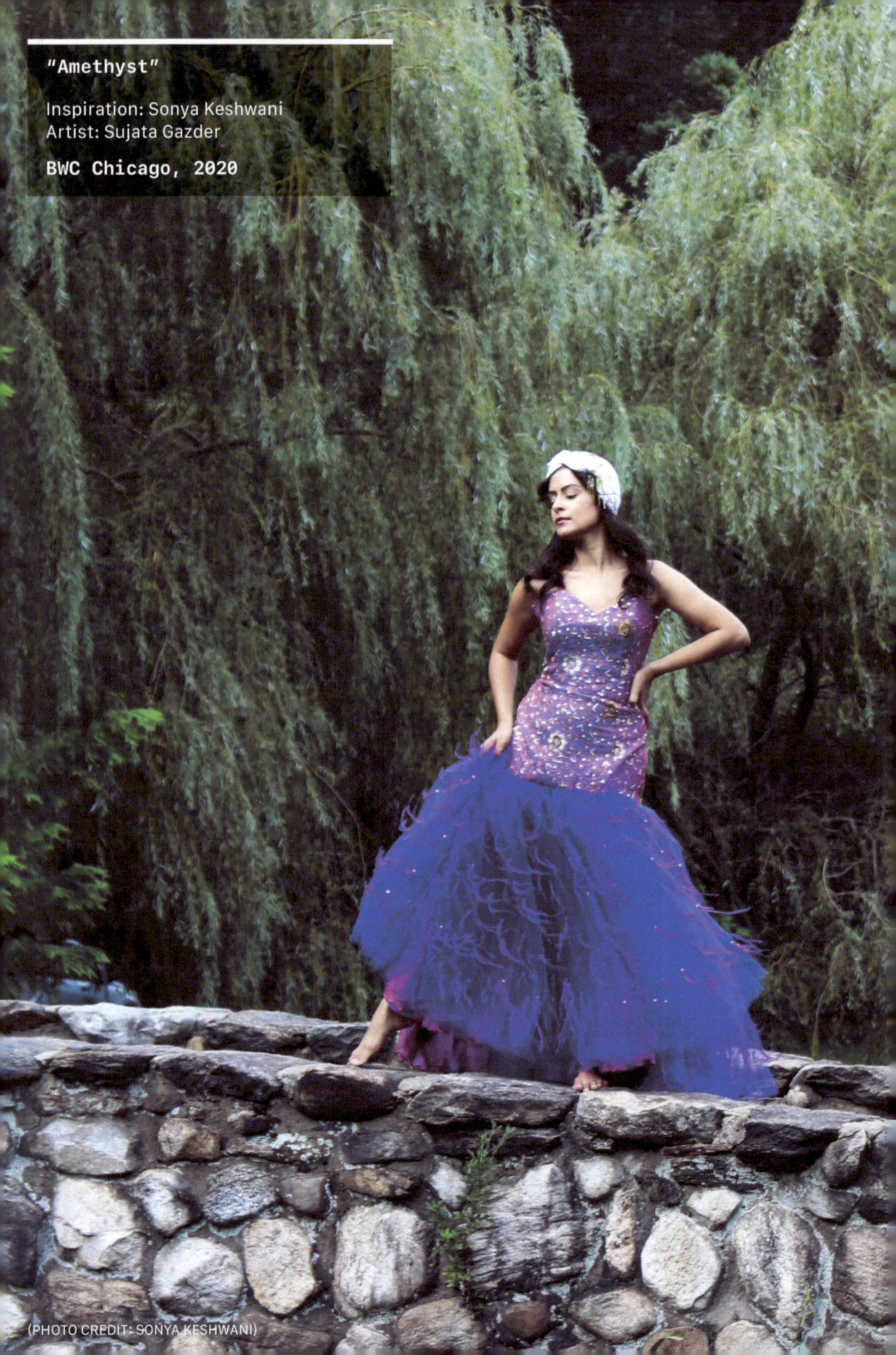

"Amethyst"

Inspiration: Sonya Keshwani
Artist: Sujata Gazder

BWC Chicago, 2020

(PHOTO CREDIT: SONYA KESHWANI)

Healing Through Fashion

While Sonya Keshwani was diagnosed with breast cancer at 29, she wasn't prepared for how hair loss can affect so many women, including herself.

"Women don't have options that make them feel beautiful and confident during hair loss," Keshwani said. "Things that are out there make you look like a cancer patient, and I wanted to look like myself."

Hair loss from cancer treatment is not just going bald – there are many side effects that go along with it, including migraines, scalp sensitivity and bruising. With the head being so sensitive during this time, wigs can be extremely uncomfortable. Additionally, there is care that comes with hair loss, including applying SPF, as well as scalp oil massages to increase blood flow.

"I wanted a small collection of beautiful head wraps and couldn't find any," Kashwani said."So I started to create my own head wraps between chemo sessions."

While in treatment, Keshwani launched her business: SyleEsteem Wardrobe. The company makes stylish head wraps that are inspired by hair loss from cancer treatment, but can be worn by anyone. Each wrap is designed by a cancer survivor and the special twist is for every head wrap purchased, Keswani donates a wrap to a cancer patient. There is also an option to sponsor a head wrap donation.

So, when Keshwani was chosen for 2020 Brushes with Cancer Chicago, it was clear she'd be a perfect match with fashion designer, Sujata Gazder.

"The first time we spoke, it was easy to connect with her and we share cultural backgrounds as well," Keshwani said. "She understood the dynamic of my situation in terms of my family being my support system. She knows what that's like in an Indian household."

As for Gazder's impression of Keshwani, she said she was blown away.

"She still has such joy for life and has become even stronger than she was," Gazder said. "You can either build yourself into a negative spiral or a positive one. At the end of the day, our essences are just looking for love and acceptance, and in Sonya's case I think she had the chutzpah to fight this battle and get where she is today."

Color and textiles are a big part of Gazder's work and for Keshwani, she carefully chose colors that represent a fighting spirit. The dress Sujata created for Sonya is a vibrant purple, which represents spirituality. Gold is threaded throughout the dress, which Gazder used to represent courage and is stylized as the Tree of Life, representing the support Keshwani received from her family.

"I was drawn to purple because it is a journey in understanding who you are when you go through a life changing experience like dealing with cancer," Gazder said. "The gold aspect is beautiful, it's got a sparkle to it, it's strength – all things I would associate with someone starting her own business and sticking her nose at cancer."

Finally, Gazder incorporated ostrich feathers all along the gown's skirt, representing plumage and hair loss.

"I felt plumage was part of her journey," she said. "I used ostrich feathers on the tulle because one thing that stood out was plumage – how women have this strong identity with their hair and whether you want to keep it or don't want to, there's a strong connection and I wanted to reflect that in the piece I made for her."

A Bedazzled Personality

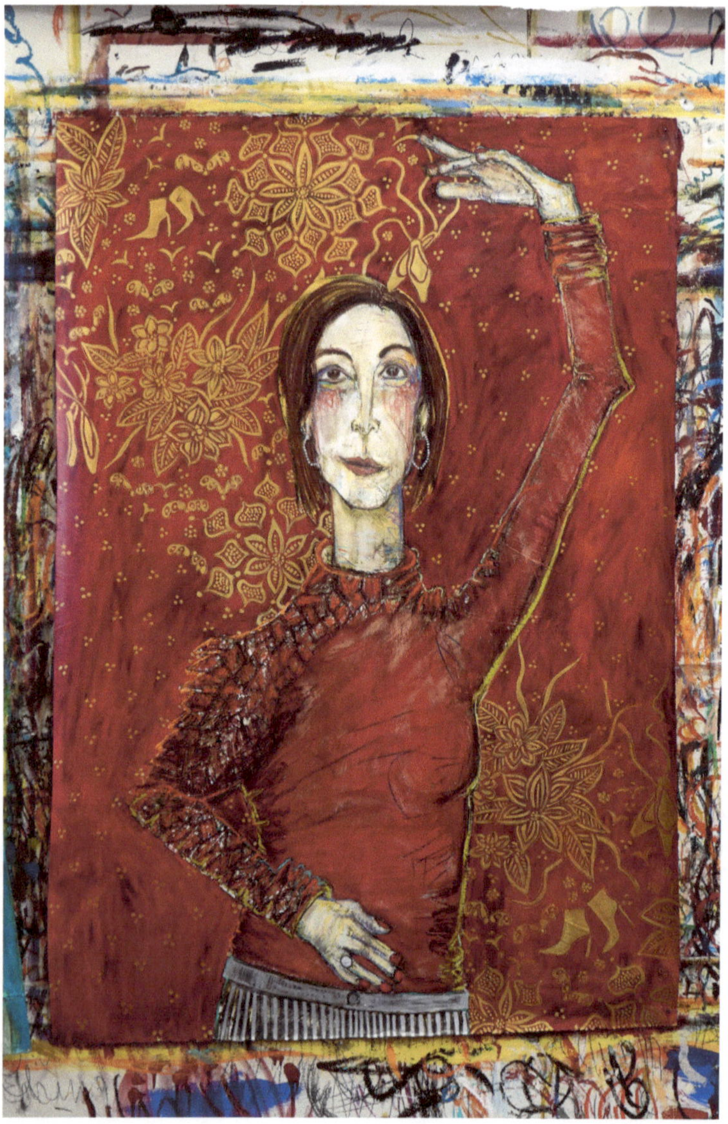

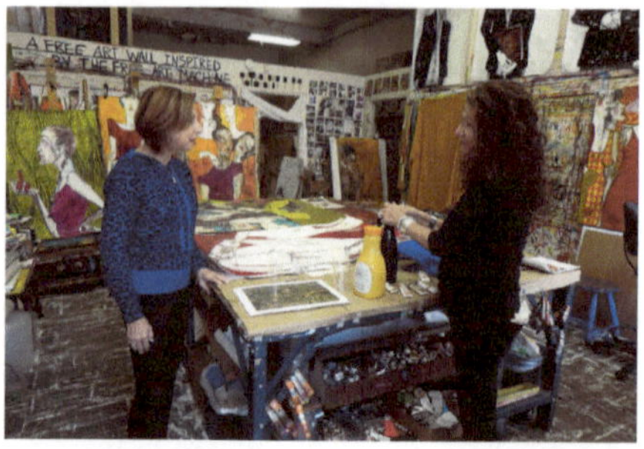

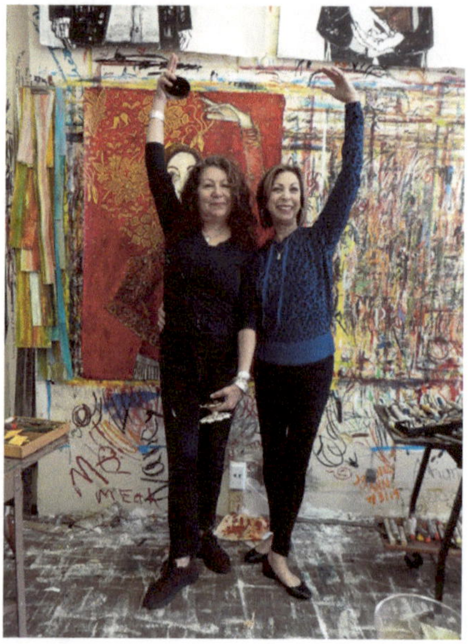

"Joni"

Inspiration: Joni Goldstein
Artist: Nancy Rosen

BWC Chicago, 2020

Total opposites often make for the best pairings, and that's what happened when Twist Out Cancer matched Inspiration Joni Goldstein and Artist Nancy Rosen.

"Joni is very bedazzled. I am not bedazzled, I am the opposite," Rosen said.

The two connected instantly and found out they have more in common than they thought. A dancer, Goldstein's happy place is the dance studio, which isn't much different from Rosen's happy place: her art studio. The duo also bonded over having sons in wrestling.

"Not often are there Jewish wrestlers," Rosen said. "Joni and I have been immersed in wrestling culture for years."

During their first meeting, they talked from 10 a.m. until 1 p.m., using that time to explore their various connections. As they got to know each other, Rosen was struck by Goldstein's bright, unique, positive attitude – an attitude that rises above the heartbreaking obstacles that were put in her path.

"Her attitude is just Joni, that's part of her story," Rosen said. "Such a great attitude and such a lovely family. It is a lot to take in but she handled it with such grace and dignity. There was never anything negative, never 'woe is me.'"

It was fall of 2004 and she was getting ready for work when she got the life-changing call from a radiologist. She said the sterile, matter-of-fact delivery made her stage 1 breast cancer diagnosis that much harder.

"I didn't know this person and it was so horrible to have someone you've never met deliver this heartbreaking news."

Goldstein immediately turned to dance. A lifelong dancer, she has been teaching at the same studio for 46 years. Even though she received one of the worst phone calls a person could get, Goldstein still had a job to do and that job got her through some of the worst days of her life.

"After I got the call, I had a four o'clock class and didn't have anyone to teach the class," she said. "So, I went there and taught ballet for a couple hours and for two hours I forgot about my diagnosis. When I got out of class I said 'This is how I'm going to live my life.'"

Goldstein was in remission when she was devastated once more. In 2016, her husband, her rock through her cancer journey, passed from Alzheimer's.

Two years after his death, her cancer came back.

"I went through my second diagnosis without my support, without my husband," she said. "But I had my family."

Friends, family and, of course, dance swooped in and helped Goldstein power through. During her second treatment, she didn't miss a single class. Like her previous cancer fight, she stocked up on colorful wigs to teach in and found comfort in sharing her diagnosis with her students.

"I went to class and told the kids that I am going to look different and one said 'My grandfather died from cancer' and another said 'My brother has cancer,'" she said. "I realized I wasn't alone and that we can do this."

For Rosen, it was important to paint a portrait of Goldstein in her natural element, showcasing all the brilliant aspects of her personality. For the portrait, Rosen asked Goldstein to bring in some props. Of course, her props were bedazzled: boots, stilettos and candles. Her pointe shoes were one of the few items not bedazzled.

In the painting, Rosen made sure to add two special items on Goldstein. One is a ring her late husband gave her during her first cancer treatment. The other is a pair of earrings she got herself for her second cancer treatment.

During the session, Goldstein posed with her arms in the air for three hours, a feat she says was no big deal.

"When I'm talking with Nancy, time just goes away," she said. "Also, when I dance, my arms go up. So, I have good strength in my arms."

The result is a bright, breathtaking portrait of a beautifully bedazzled Goldstein in her happy place.

"She got the essence of me," Goldstein said. "I'm very easy to read and she got it all. What you see is me. I'm just here."

Not only is Goldstein's journey immortalized in Rosen's painting, but so is their special relationship.

"Our connection was brought out in her painting," Goldstein said. "Nancy is artistic in her own way and I'm part of that signature now."

"In 1987, when I was 6 months old, I was diagnosed with a rare type of Neuroblastoma. I underwent countless chemotherapy and radiation treatments for 2.5 years. Round after round, I was a sweet smiling baby undergoing intensive treatments in the form of "adult" doses.

I'm a cancer survivor, but I feel that my "Coping with cancer" story belongs mainly to my beloved parents, who courageously fought my cancer for me. Their coping with my cancer is the first and most important life-lesson I have ever learned: Never to lose hope, and to always think positive and fight hard until overcoming the obstacle.

Being privileged to survive the cancer keeps me in proportion all the time, and makes me appreciate and enjoy every minute of every day. I'm thankful for everything I have, and I always aspire to have the fullest and the most interesting life while I live.

Before I beat it, my cancer injured my spinal cord so I remained paralyzed in my lower body, and as someone who had to learn how to fight for her life even before learning how to walk, I grew up to be a strong social activist and a justice fighter for accessibility and integration of people with disabilities in different fields of life.

Naturally, my life-mission has become to help people to cope with their own personal struggles and to remind them that in life - It's better to learn how to dance in the rain, than to wait for the storm to pass!"

—VITAL ZINGER, INSPIRATION

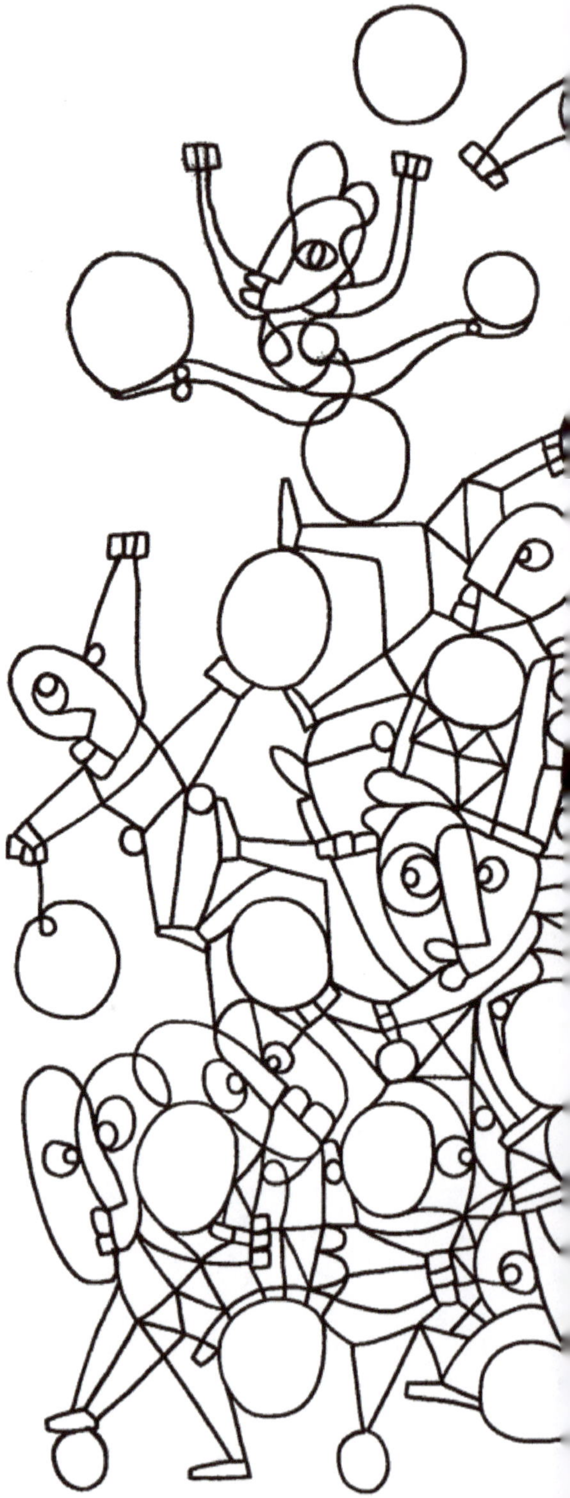

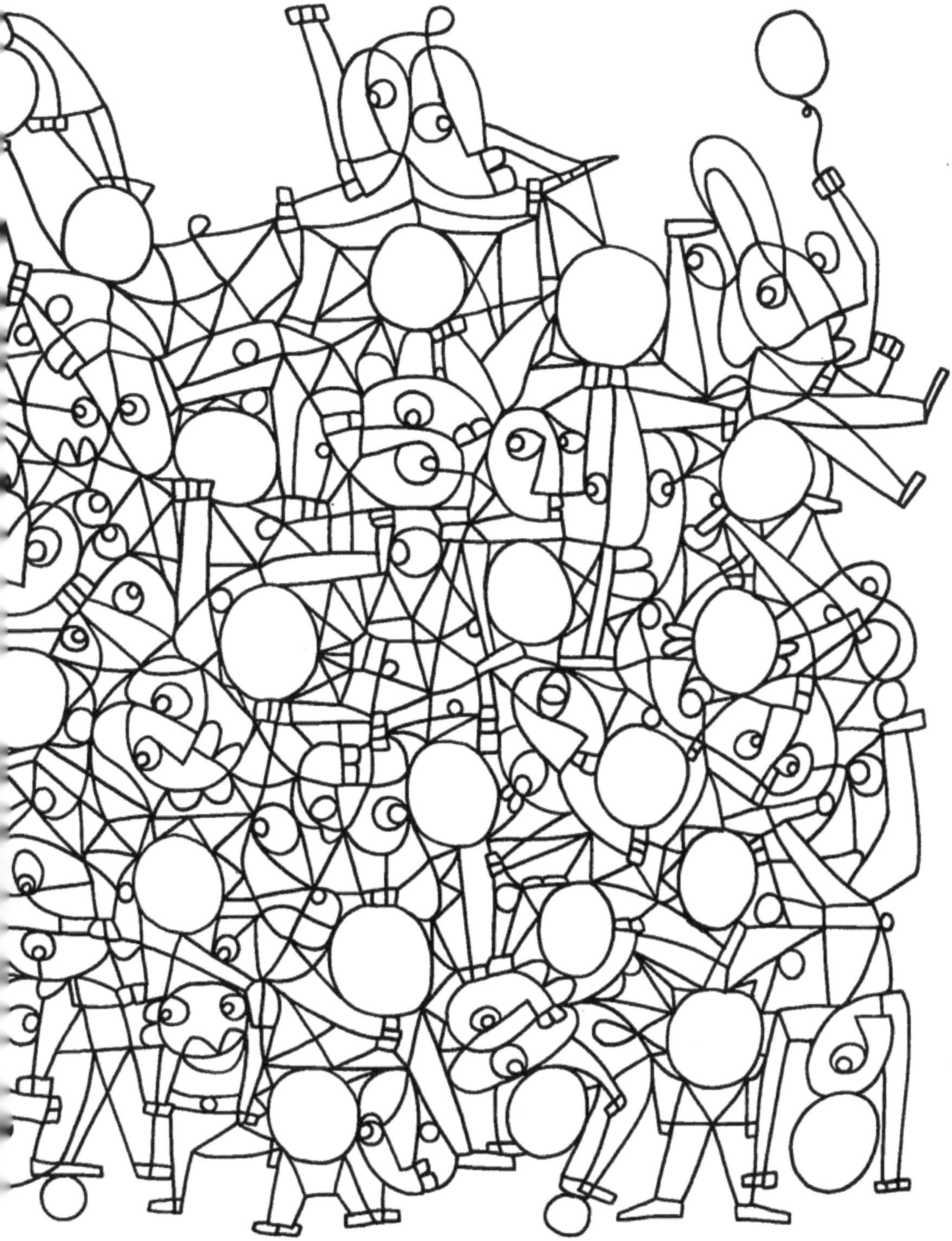

"What if Everyone Was Just Like Me"

Inspiration: Vital Zinger
Artist: Nissim Ben Aderet

BWC Tel Aviv, 2018

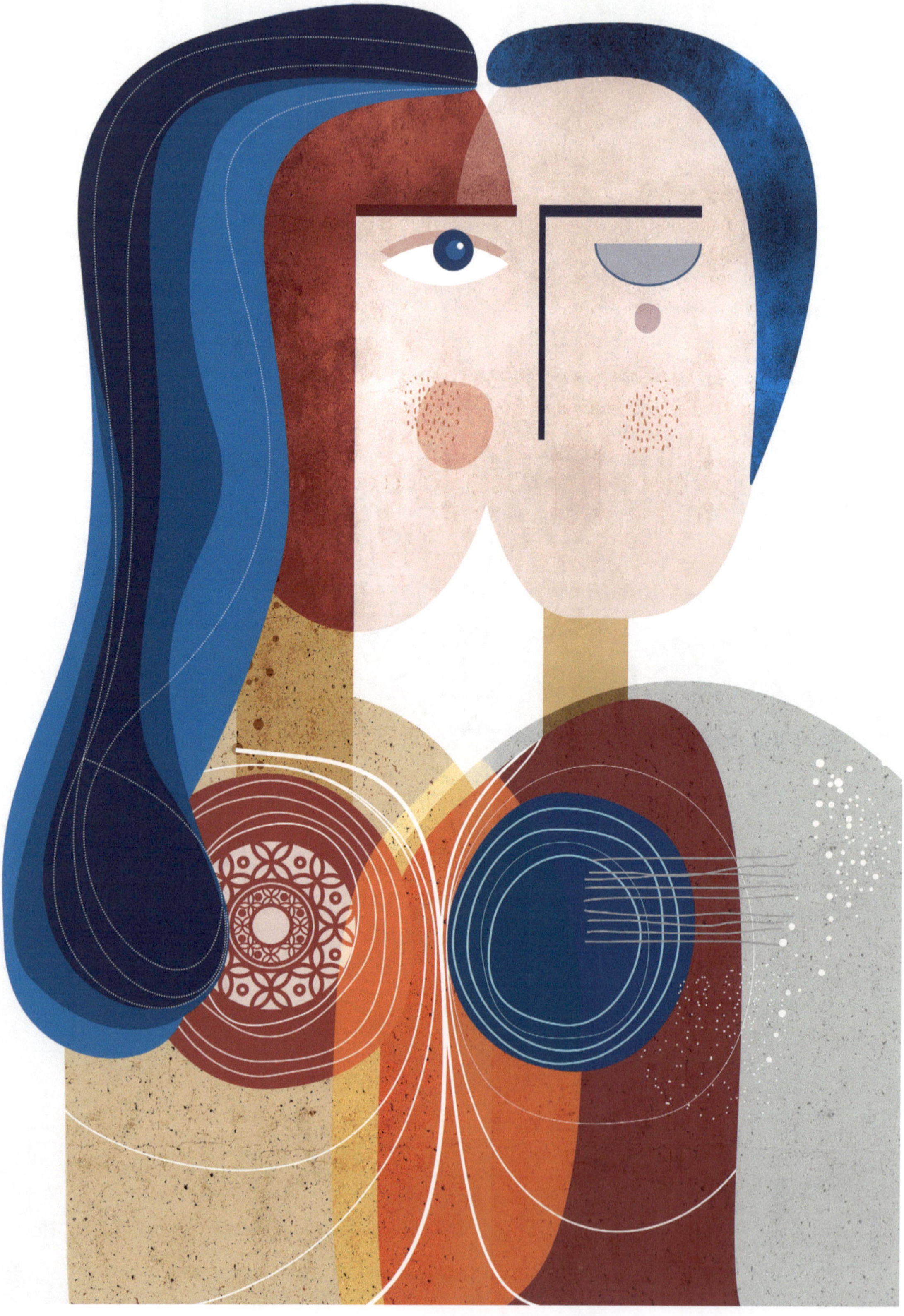

"I watched my mother fight this disease for almost 20 years before passing away from it. When it came for me, a mere 3 years later, I took a completely different treatment approach: guns a-blazing, and I left no stone unturned so that I would be cancerfree for a long, long time."

—VIRGINIA CHAMPOUX-SOKOLOFF,
SURVIVOR & CAREGIVER

"Our Tangled Stories is the story of Virginia and her late husband Jay, which are completely intertwined. While Virginia was battling a deadly and rapidly spreading breast cancer, double mastectomy and its intense aftermath, her husband underwent lung failure and passed away, leaving her with two young children, and a tremendous fight to battle. Layered and complex, her story had so many levels. The center point of the story is the breast and the lung. The place where it all began. The breast and the lungs are generally in the same area of the body and I tried to show how where one began and one ended. Their stories are tangled, interlinked and can be seen as two breasts, one breast and a lung or two lungs. The radiating lines tangle and weave the stories together. The tattoos on the breast that Virginia chose to cover up the scars is symbolically represented, while the hair also plays a big part in the composition. While Jay is no longer present physically, he is still a big part of the story in spirit and so the closed eye, the lines and dots that symbolize his onward journey. I deliberately kept away from black, choosing instead shades of blue, rust, terracotta and flesh tones. The female form representing Virginia is strong, vibrant and is an inspiration to look up to. I have had to fight tears every time I worked on it. The magnitude of what she had to go through was staggering. The statement I am trying to make through this art piece is both poignant, harsh yet strong and determined. A celebration of who Virginia is and the optimism with which she has forged on. Getting to know her, her sense of humor and the tenacity with which she fought the biggest battle of her life was a gift to me. If ever faced with this kind of adversity, her strength is what I hope to imbibe in my own life."

—ISHITA BANERJEE, ARTIST

"Our Tangled Stories"

Inspiration: Virginia Champoux
Artist: Ishita Banerjee

BWC Montreal, 2018

Finding Community

One day, Twist Out Cancer Founder and CEO Jenna Benn Shersher came across a viral video of Rena Williams and knew she had to reach out.

You see, Rena has a story very similar to Jenna's.

When she was diagnosed with triple-negative breast cancer, Rena turned to dance as a way to manage her diagnosis and treatment.

"I needed a way to escape," she said. "I've always been an athletic person, so I knew it had to be something moving my body. And I love finding comfort in music."

In order to attack the cancer, Rena needed 16 rounds of chemotherapy – an intimidating and exhausting amount of sessions. Through dance, she tackled each round at a time by learning a choreographed dance leading up to the session and performing the number after she completed each chemo treatment.

"I would come home from work, practice a dance and by the time I was done, I was so exhausted I would fall asleep."

Up most nights with anxiety over her diagnosis and treatment, dance finally gave Rena the rest she needed.

But it was the last day of treatment that would change her life. On that day, her coworkers surprised her with a flash mob.

"We're dancing for you," they told her.

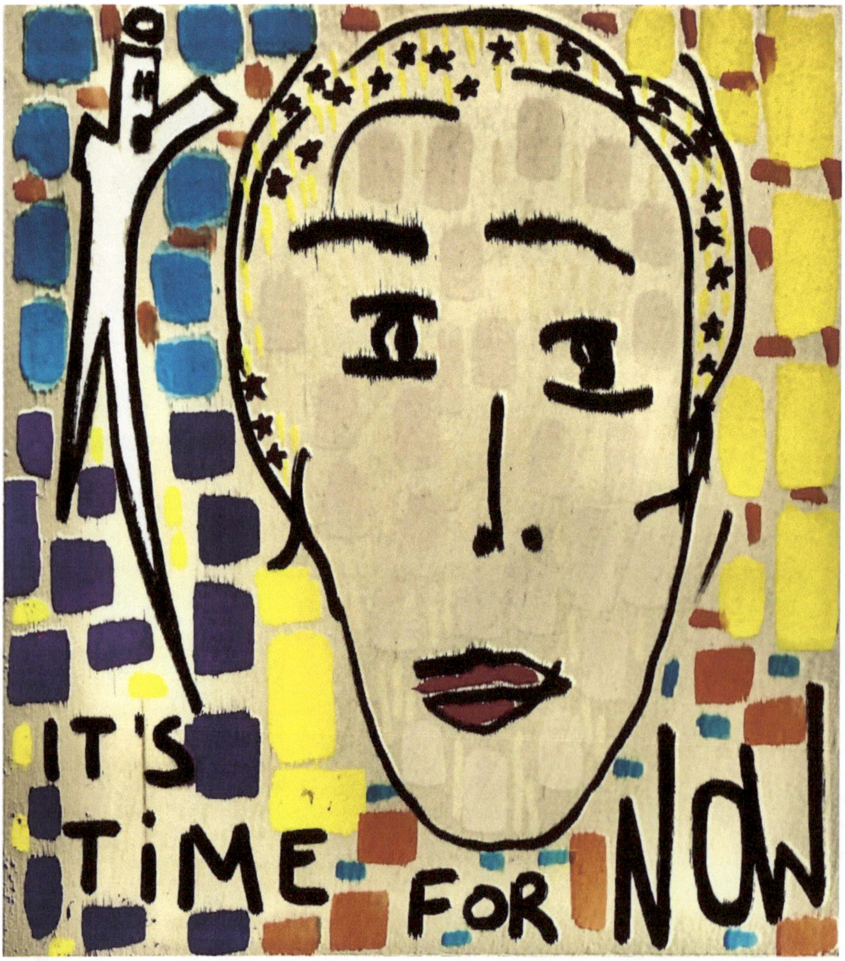

"Rena"

Inspiration: Rena Williams
Artist: Murielle Cohen

BWC Austin, 2022

The act of kindness went viral and eventually made its way to Jenna, who reached out to Rena.

"When I learned about Rena's story, I just knew I needed to reach out to her," Jenna said. "Her spirit, her tenacity, and her zest for life was infectious. I just knew that Twist would be a wonderful fit for her, and we are so grateful she is now deeply immersed in our community."

"You need to live in the moment, live right now"

—RENA WILLIAMS

Compared to other Brushes with Cancer Inspirations, Rena's pairing was unique. She was paired with Artist Murielle Cohen, who showed Rena new perspectives and a signature portrait style.

"It was neat because she lives in Israel and our lives are so different," Rena said. "Sometimes, it's good to have your eyes opened up to how someone else lives when it's different from your life."

When Rena met Murielle, she was in the radiation portion of treatment and kept thinking of the future.

"Radiation is such a weird time in the treatment schedule," Rena said. "I was so close to being done and having weird feelings like 'Now what am I going to do? I just sit around and see what happens?'"

From an ocean away, Murielle helped comfort Rena during this strange time by helping to bring her back to the present.

"In all our conversations, what kept coming back was 'You need to live in the moment, live right now,'" Rena said. "I needed to hear that because I was living in the future and worrying what would happen. Right now, the sun's out, there are flowers that are blooming and I could miss all of that."

Murielle's specialty is 30-second portraits, which she was introduced to by a friend. At the time, Murielle was living in New York City and working as a model. When the city experienced the horrors of September 11, Murielle utilized these portraits to help her community heal. Carrying a pad of paper and black pen, she'd walk up to people and ask to draw their portrait. When she was finished, they kept the piece as a gift. She used this same gift to help Rena's healing.

"I was really happy when she chose the 30-second portrait format, because that's her and what she loves to do the most."

In April of this year, Rena celebrated one year of no cancer evidence. Naturally, she had a disco-themed dance party to celebrate. She brought the same enthusiasm to the Brushes with Cancer virtual event, turning her home into a red-carpet event and donning her favorite formalwear.

"I feel like I have been brought into this family, and the more I heal, the more I'm able to give. The Twist Out Cancer community has already given me so much that I can't wait to grow this relationship and give back."

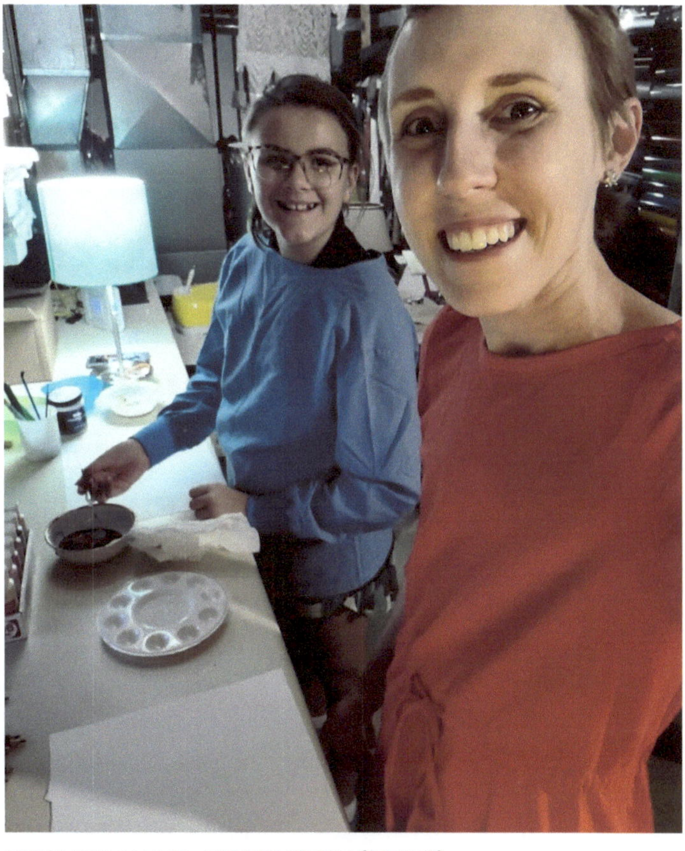

RENA WILLIAMS, INSPIRATION (RIGHT)

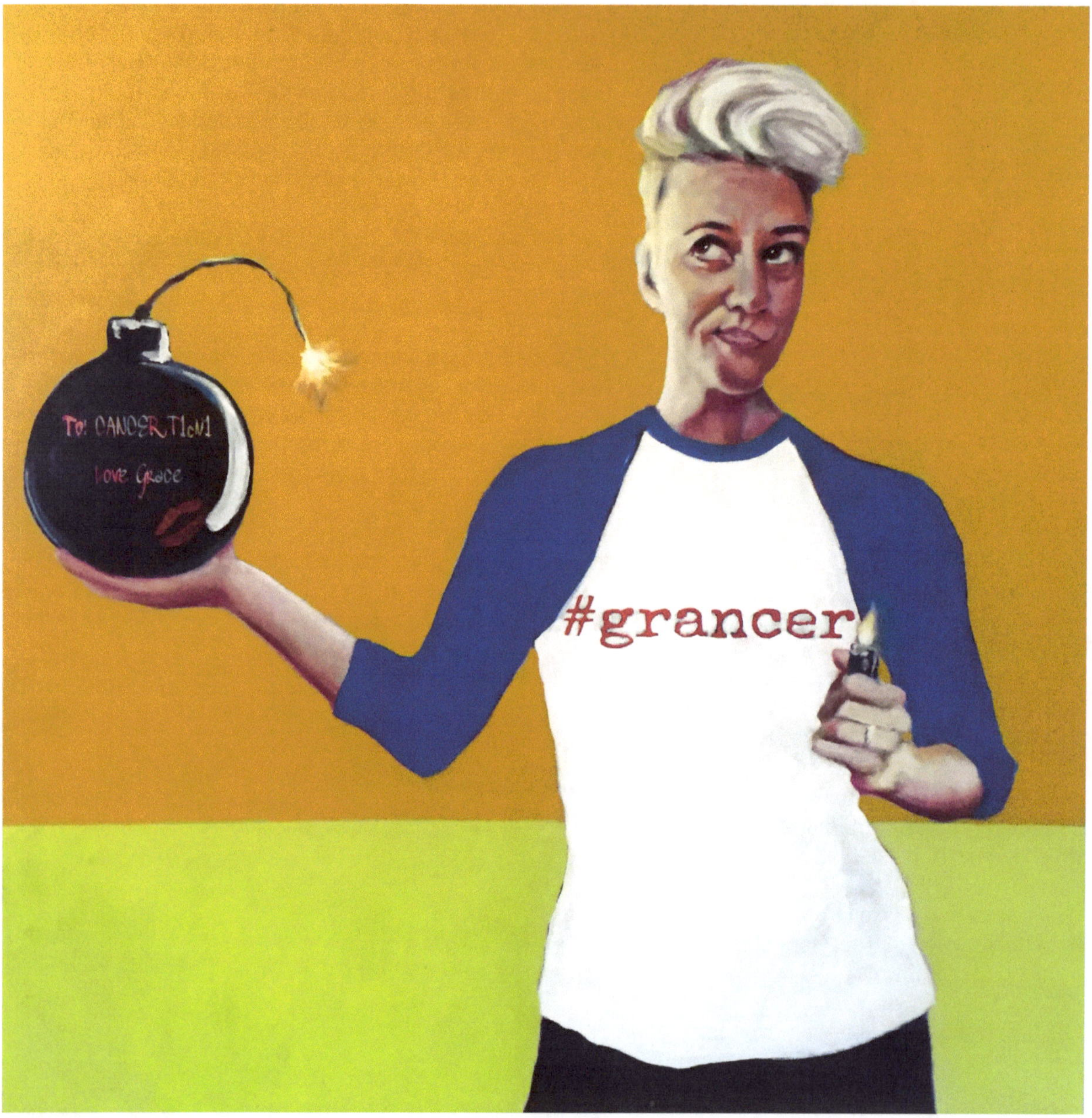

"Bombs Away"

Inspiration: Grace Fauls Lombardo
Artist: Bowen Kline

BWC Chicago, 2017

"I was diagnosed with stage 2a non-BRCA breast cancer as a very healthy, 35 year-old mother of 3 small children. After my cancer diagnosis, everything happened so quickly. Within weeks, I had a bilateral mastectomy and a subsequent second surgery to remove more nodes. Next came a nasty infection followed by 12 weeks of chemotherapy and reconstructive surgery.

Through it all, there were a few constants that helped me traverse my 'year of cancer.' First was the overwhelming love and support of my family and friends, most notably my sister, Jennie. She stopped her life to keep me alive. She cared for me so tenderly and meticulously. The closeness we cultivated is a lucky byproduct of the disease. In the very early days after diagnosis, my sister encouraged me to start a blog, a way to keep family and friends within the loop. What started as a way to disseminate information, turned into something much larger. Blogging about my experiences and feelings gave me an outlet I had no idea I needed. True to my nature, I was extremely open and honest in my writing and though I was walking through fire, I managed to infuse each entry with humor, which was part storytelling and part coping mechanism. Through the power of sharing and the internet, my blog grew exponentially. Since inception, my blog has had over 130,000 visitors. The impact I have been able to have on strangers who have been touched by a cancer odyssey is truly a gift."

—GRACE FAULS LOMBARDO, INSPIRATION

"I would like to introduce everyone to Amazing Grace Fauls Lombardo. A year ago, she was given unexpected and unwelcome news that she had been diagnosed with breast cancer. This was shocking, because she believed herself to be healthy and energetically pursuing her life with her family. To help cope with this distressing news, Grace began to write. And write she did! She started her blog, Grancer, a playful mash-up of Grace and cancer, as a way to describe her feelings during this terrible time. She spoke of pain and anger as well as finding humor. It was her writing that broke her through her depression."

—BOWEN KLINE, ARTIST

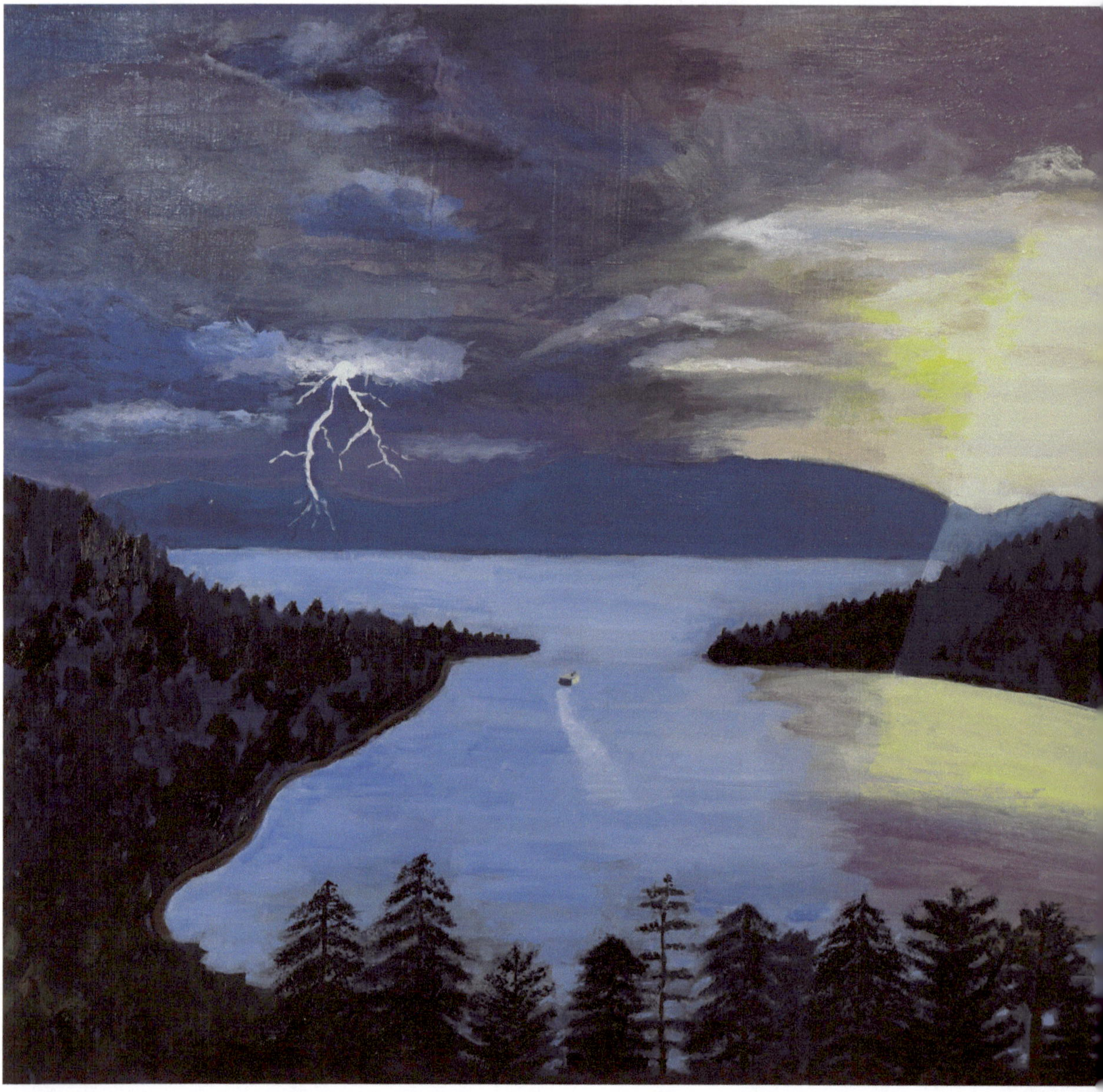

"Storm Receding - Sunlight Beckons"

Inspiration: Sarah Wartell
Artist: Judy Abplanalp

BWC Southwest, 2022

"On average, one out of 20 individuals are impacted by colon cancer. It is the second leading cause of cancer-related deaths. These statistics aren't meant to frighten you - but they do mean to serve as a wakeup call of how common this disease really is. The good news is because of research, there are over a million survivors alive in the U.S. presently. In my particular case, being young, thin framed, with perfect lab results and in my early 40s didn't help my doctors reach a diagnosis in a timely fashion. Procedures like colonoscopies don't often get ordered unless you are 45. That investigative surgery saved my life by finding the mass. Symptoms alone can't diagnose cancer, even as horrible as they are. Consult with your physician if you are exhibiting any and keep advocating for yourself. You know your body best, listen to what your guts says and take action. It could save your life!"

—SARAH WARTELL, INSPIRATION

"I first learned about Brushes with Cancer from my son, who participated as an Artist in last year's program. At the time I decided to apply, we were all in the midst of the pandemic. My usual challenges, supplied by piano groups and oil painting classes, had been cut off, and I was more open to the very challenging opportunity offered by Brushes with Cancer than I would have been under other circumstances. I felt I could combine my skills as a psychologist with the chance to get to know and perhaps be helpful to someone dealing with cancer.

Sarah, my Inspiration, and I, visited a number of times via Facetime, and it was during those conversations that I learned about her background, her interests and her many talents. That was also how I learned about her experience with cancer and what it has meant to her.

I made an initial attempt in a drawing to combine a large number of ideas into what I imagined would be my eventual painting. However, despite multiple attempts, there was just too much material. So, I decided I would focus on the environment Sarah had described as being central to her life — water and mountains. The painting depicts a scene around Lake Tahoe, one of Sarah's favorite places. The lightning storm is ending; the sunbeams are drawing the boat (containing Sarah) to the light, which represents a bright future."

—JUDY ABPLANALP, ARTIST

"Cancer for me - as it is with most survivors - was a life changing experience. I never knew how strong I was until I had to deal with the challenges of chemotherapy, radiation and a major cancer surgery. And by strong, that includes physical, emotional, and spiritual strength. I had time during treatment for much introspection on my life, and was able to reconcile and forgive myself for the questionable choices of my youth. I had been holding a lot of those in my heart for a long time, and needed to finally let go of the past. I came to a greater faith and trust in God for His plan for my life. Spending so much time in the hospital during treatment, I became acutely aware of the need for patient support and advocacy in the cancer community, and hope to dedicate time to supporting my brother and sister warriors as soon as I retire in January (yay!!) Physically, cancer may have saved my life! For many years, I struggled with weight challenges, and knew that it would catch up with me eventually in heart problems, or something else life threatening. During the course of treatment I lost 120 pounds, wwhich probably saved me from a potential heart attack. Yin and Yang...good and bad. I was really sick, but it saved my life."

—BOBBIE TIEDT DONOHEW, INSPIRATION

"My wonderful Inspiration, Bobbie, provided me with photos and CT scans of her cancer and scars. This painting is my re-interpretation of the CT scan of her neck, with the cancer in jewel tones. My goal was to create an image of beauty abstracted from the medical imagery of Bobbie's tumor in the hopes of giving her a treasured souvenir with which to remember her inspiring story of survival from cancer. I hope this work offers Bobbie a fraction of the inspiration she has given me in sharing her cancer story with me!"

—KATHRYN TUBBS, ARTIST

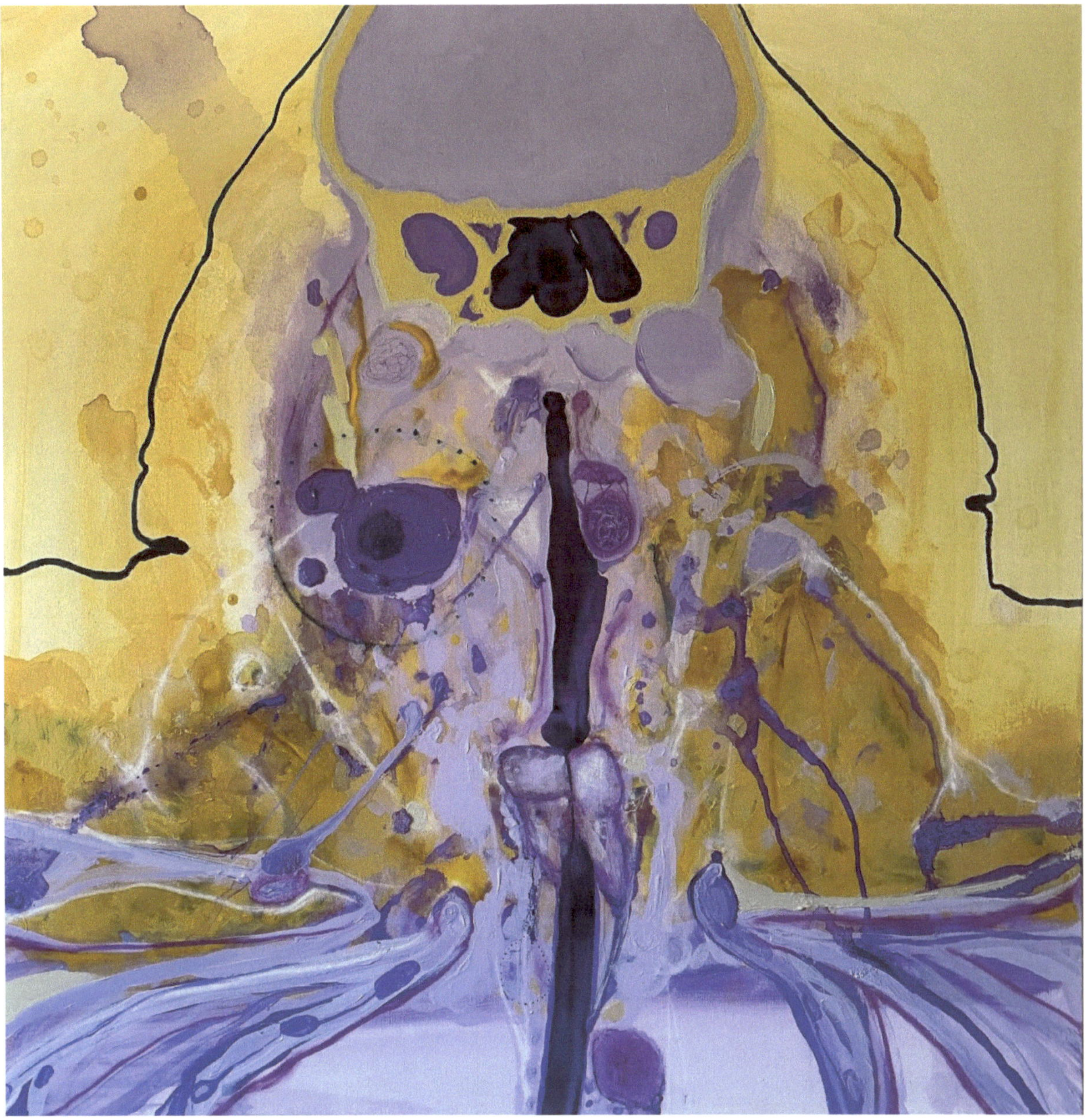

"She Overcame Everything Meant to Destroy Her"

Inspiration: Bobbie Tiedt Donohew
Artist: Kathryn Tubbs

BWC Northeast, 2021

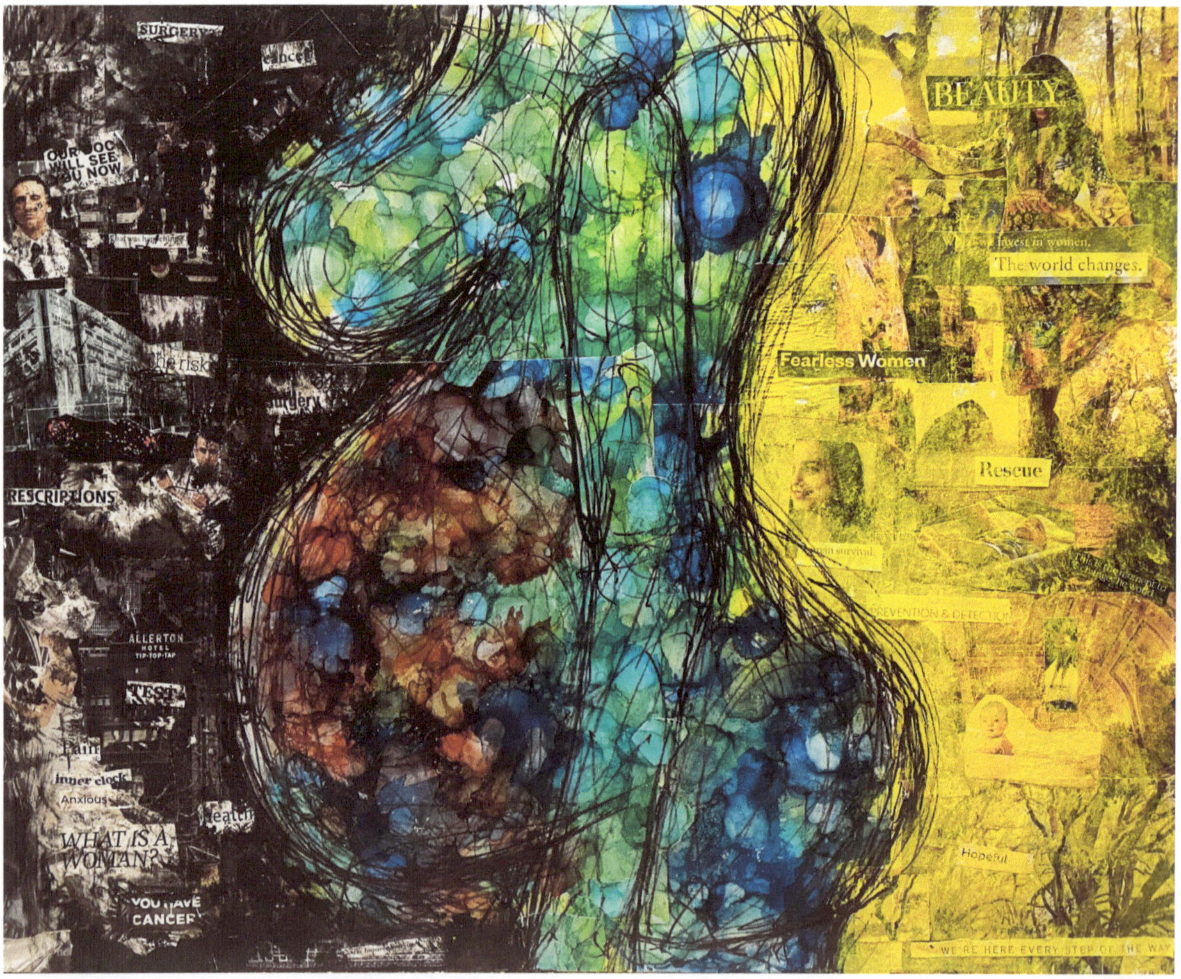

"Expecting"

Inspiration: Soraya Fata
Artist: Shefali Khanna

BWC Midwest, 2021

Life After Cancer

WRITTEN BY SORAYA FATA

It's May again, a time to celebrate motherhood; a month full of Mother's Day-themed events, promotions and social media posts of mamas with their little ones. I tap into my inner strength and somehow manage to ward off the onslaught of messages with the protective shield I've built up over the years.

Every once in a while though, something penetrates my outer layer and pierces my heart. It's usually a photo, not one of those posed ones, but a candid shot perfectly capturing a mother's love for her child or a family shot celebrating the fundamental life experience of parenthood. On a rational level, I know these photos aren't meant to highlight what I don't have in my life, but on an emotional level, I can't help but feel inadequate. I've yearned for motherhood for so long now, but year after year, my desire has gone unfulfilled. For me, Mother's Day is just a reminder of my pain, of my story of cancer and infertility.

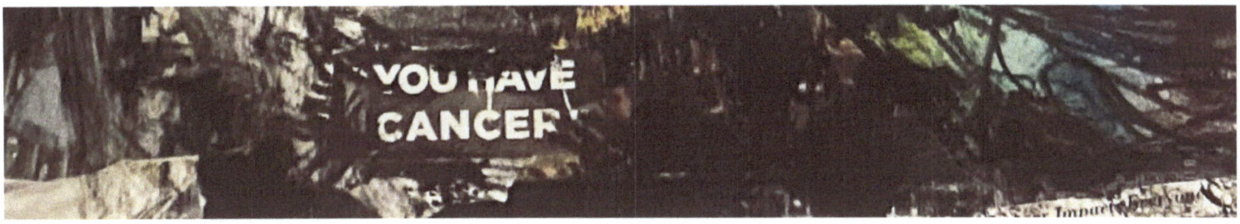

OVARIAN CANCER AND INFERTILITY

I met my husband in my late 30s, but we hoped there was still time to start a family. We didn't wait long to consult fertility specialists, given my age. In the summer of 2018, my fertility doctor noticed a mass on my right ovary. We were hopeful that it was nothing, maybe just a cyst.

But several months later, it was confirmed to be a rare form of ovarian cancer. During surgery to remove that ovary, another mass was found on my other ovary. Though a full hysterectomy is protocol, the doctor conducting the surgery was aware of my desire to have children, and therefore, removed only the mass on the left ovary and a portion of tissue around it. I was left with a small area of ovarian tissue, as well as my uterus.

I was warned that when the final pathology report came back, I might need chemotherapy, radiation or another operation to remove the rest of my reproductive system. Additionally, the scar tissue on my left ovary made conceiving naturally unlikely because it might block the release of eggs. The best option was IVF, which I had already been through twice by then. The invasive and expensive process required me to inject myself with hormones several times a day, leaving me constantly ill and unable to fully participate in life. I struggled to balance work and medical appointments and was forced to pay out of pocket for the procedures, since my health insurance didn't cover the costs.

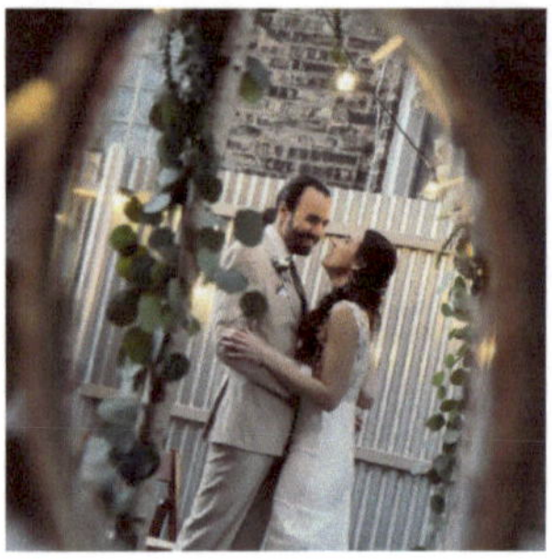

Each round felt like a rollercoaster, which started full of hope and desires for our future as a family, but inevitably ended in disappointment. I felt inadequate as a woman and as a partner, though my husband tried to convince me the contrary was true. I went through round after round of IVF, eventually totaling eight rounds. My chances of conceiving were slim, given what little ovarian tissue I had remaining.

People close to me urged me to let go of the idea of motherhood and accept my life circumstances. I tried to remind myself how lucky I was that we caught the cancer early, that I didn't have to go through radiation or chemotherapy like so many other cancer survivors.

Despite moments of real gratitude, I struggled to detach my story of infertility from my cancer diagnosis, given how tightly they were interwoven. Even though I survived cancer, I hadn't yet survived infertility.

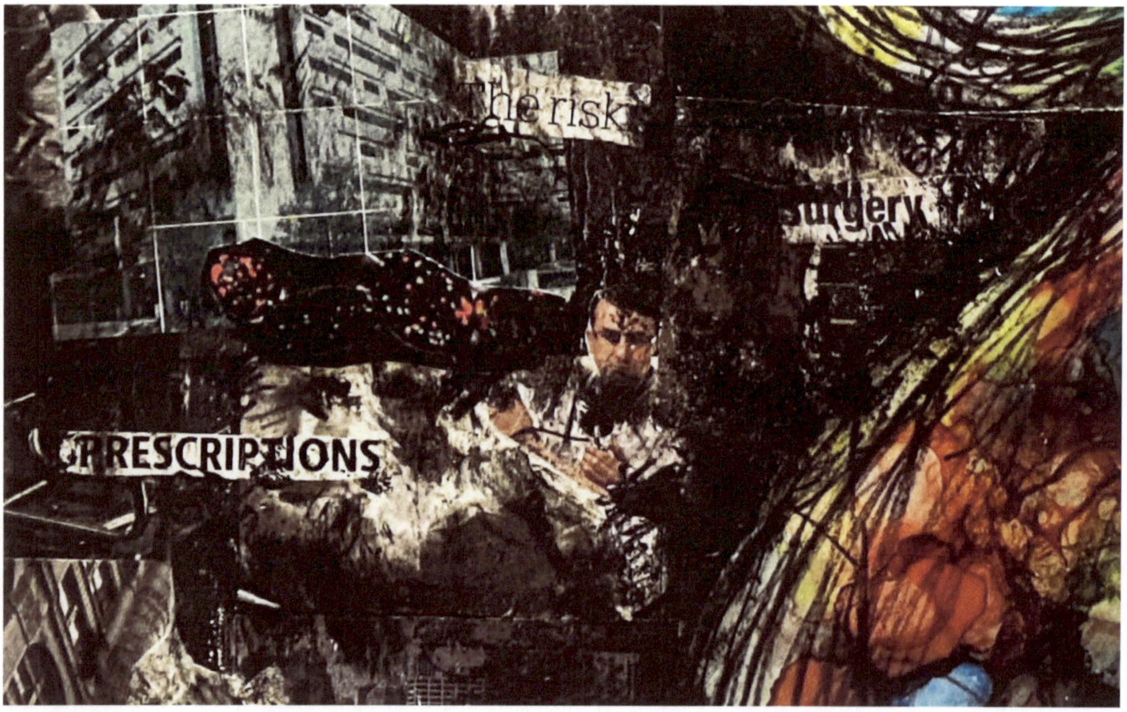

ART AS AN EMOTIONAL OUTLET

My husband is a professional jazz musician and during this painful period in our life together, I was always envious that he could lose himself in his art, express his emotions through music and deal with the situation in that way. My legal career didn't offer me the same emotional outlet.

When a good friend told me about Brushes with Cancer, I knew immediately I wanted to participate. I didn't know what would come of it, but I hoped the experience would bring me clarity and an opportunity to reflect on my experience with cancer. Although it's only been a few months since meeting the artist and mentor I will work with this year, what I've discovered so far is that sharing my experience with illness to those willing to listen is powerful. Even more powerful is the process of turning that experience into art.

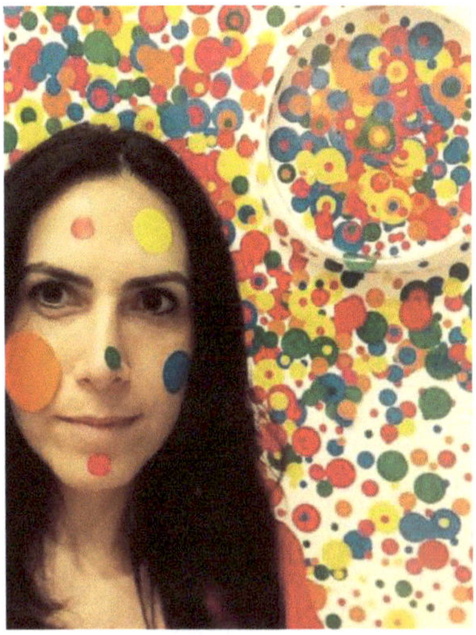

Illness is something that feels completely out of our hands, but taking our story and giving it texture and color, helps us seize back the control over our story. It's like flipping the script. We decide how we want the world to see our story versus the world deciding how to see our story.

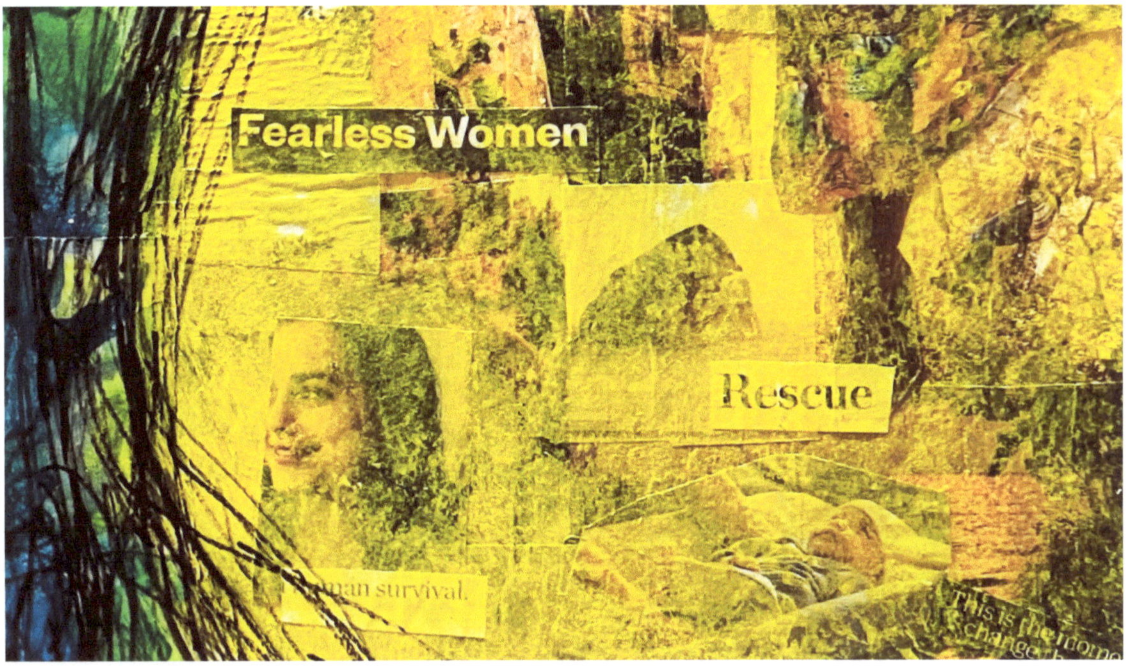

A TIME TO HEAL

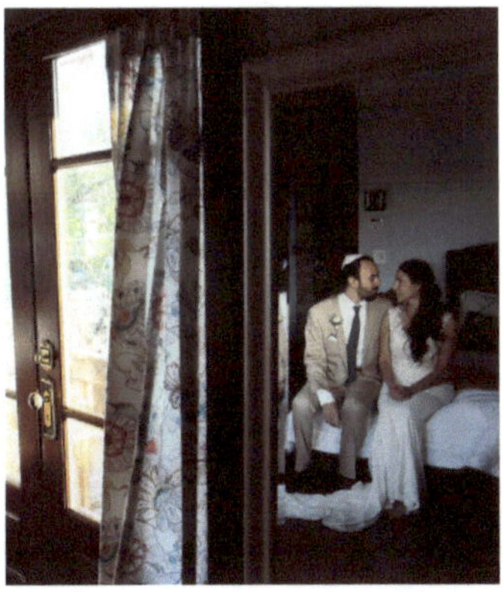

This year, I can finally begin to heal from the past.

As I continue to share my story with my artist and mentor and with others in the Brushes with Cancer community, I feel a sense of lightness. It's as if this weight that I was carrying around for years, this grief, is suddenly lifting from me.

I'm healing for another reason, too.

This year, I'm beyond grateful to find that there's a life forming inside of me, proving that sometimes if we're persistent and lucky enough, there is life after cancer.

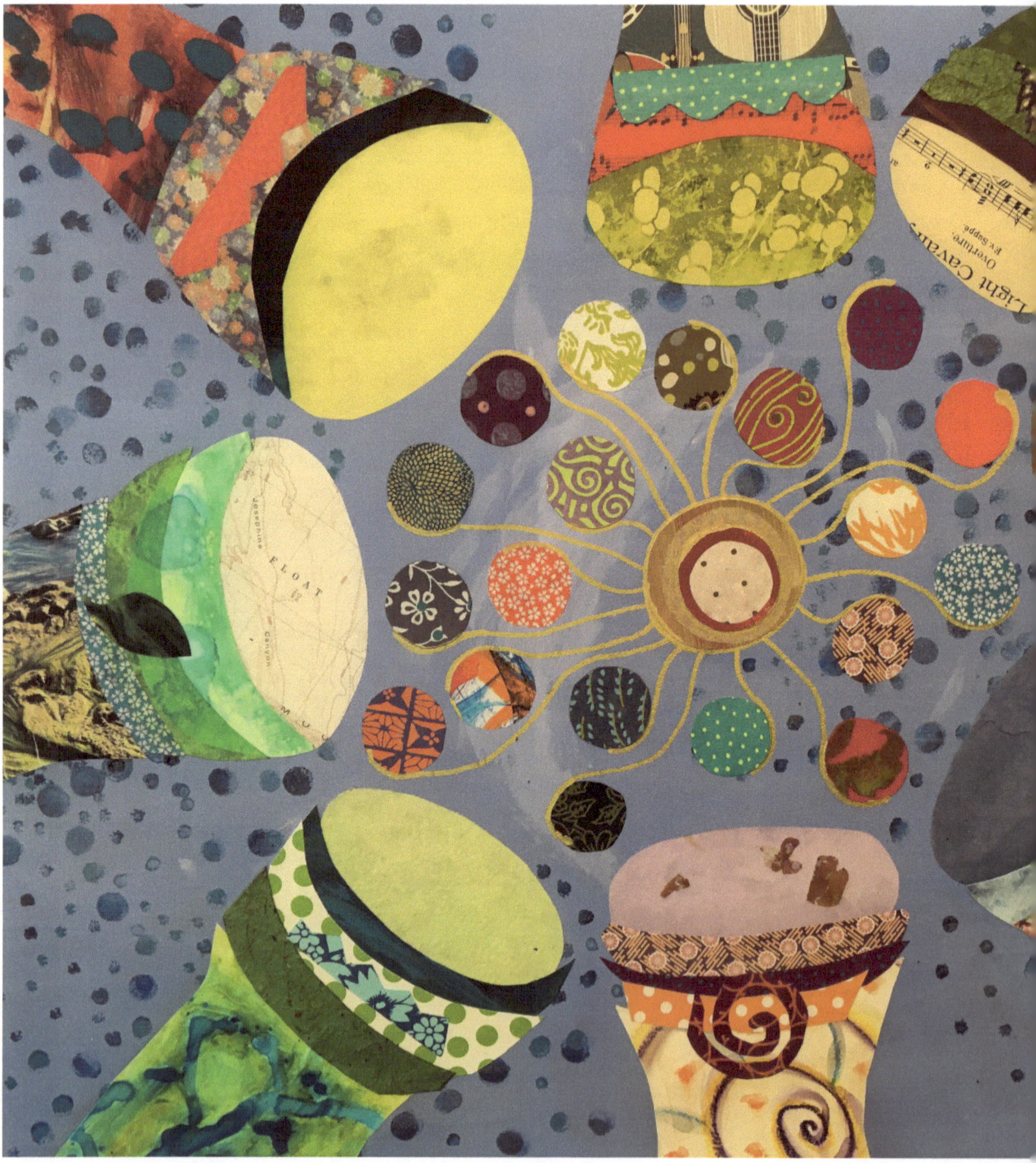

"Connecting Rhythms"

Inspiration: Noah Plotkin
Artist: Mignon Dupepe

BWC Midwest, 2021

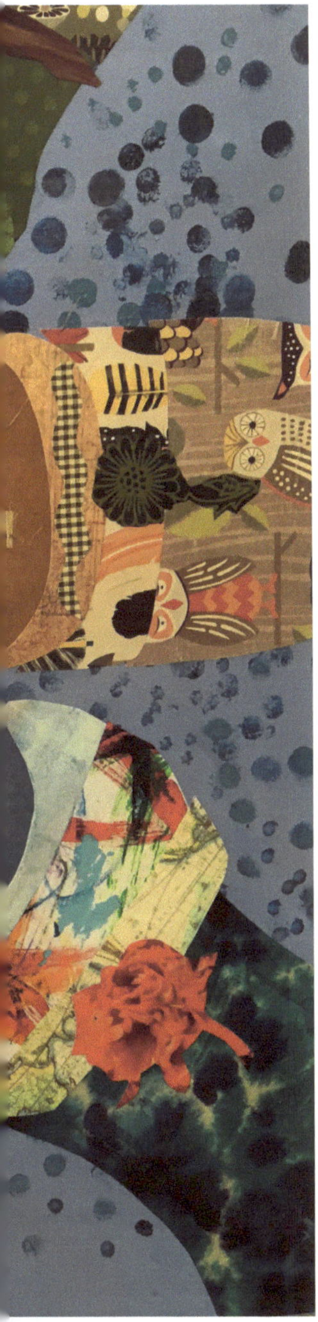

I learned many lessons and tricks through my road to recovery and I feel like there isn't enough room here with the word count to explain it all. So, I am open and available to anyone who has any questions about R-CHOP Chemotherapy, Lymphoma of the Pelvic Bone, pain management, etc. What I can share briefly is (CBD and THC RSO Oil helped immensely) Cannabis in general was a huge wellness factor for me. That and diet. Plant proteins, green juices and smoothies daily! I am happy to speak about my experience at any time.

—NOAH PLOTKIN, INSPIRATION

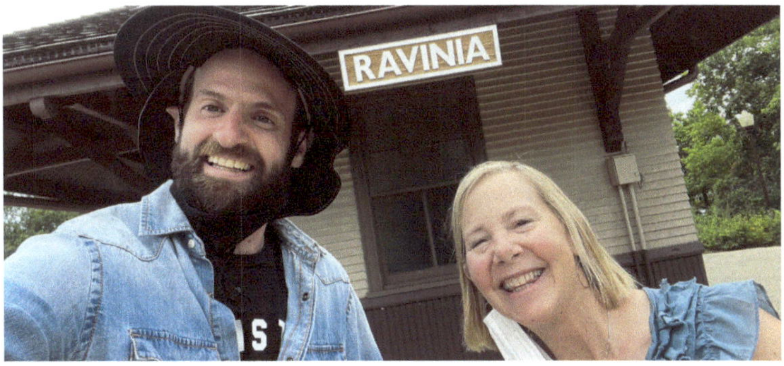

NOAH PLOTKIN & MIGNON DUPEPE

"While my Inspiration, Noah Plotkin, is a talented drummer, percussionist, artist, wellness advocate, and event organizer, he is also a compassionate husband, friend, and family supporter. Ultimately, Noah is an incredible connector. His passion for using music for healing, good health, wellness, and for building strong communities is demonstrated by his work with Life Rhythms, and his collaborations with Living Whole Online, Nora's Project, and Brushes with Cancer (Inspiration and an Artist this year). In addition, Noah coordinates live music for Congregation Am Shalom and local farmer's markets throughout Chicago.

Noah's music practice of using drum circles to soothe worries, inspire self-expression, reestablish healthy life rhythms, and unite people inspired the art piece. The healing drum circle as a metaphor for a community with individuals of many beliefs and backgrounds coming together to share in a vision of healing and growth captured Noah's spirit and story brilliantly.

Noah's diffuse b-cell lymphoma of his pelvic bone did not stop him from continuing to build and support connections this year. These b-cells (a community of cells) are displayed subtly behind the bold and colorful collaged drum circle. Each drum represents a unique piece of Noah's story. My wish is for this drum circle to empower Noah and the viewer in the act of celebrating community and life."

—MIGNON DUPEPE, ARTIST

"Find Your Light"

Inspiration: Jackie Herigodt
Artist: Jeff Guerrero

BWC Midwest, 2021

SURVIVOR
FIGHTER
LOVE
HOPE
HEALING
BREATHE
CONNECTION
WHY
FUCK CANCER
HELPING OTHERS

CONTINUED >

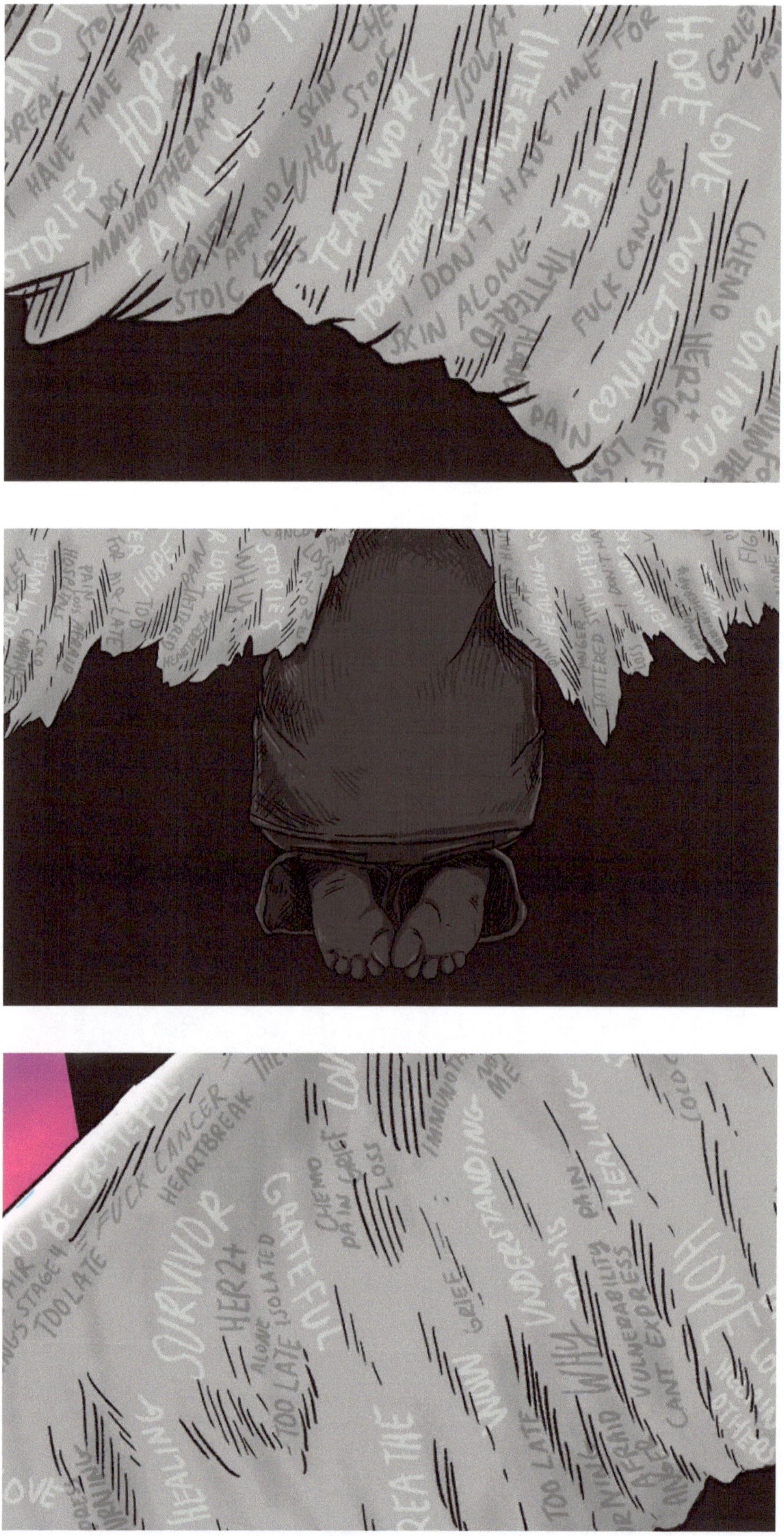
HOPE
STORIES
FAMILY
IMMUNOTHERAPY
AFRAID
STOIC
WHY
TEAM WORK
TOGETHERNESS
ISOLATION
I DON'T HAVE TIME FOR
SKIN ALONE
TATTERED
FIGHTER
FUCK CANCER
PAIN CONNECTION
HER2+
GRIEF
LOSS
LOVE
CHEMO
SURVIVOR
TOO LATE
HEARTBREAK
HEALING
GRATEFUL
ALONE
ISOLATED
UNDERSTANDING
VULNERABILITY
CANT EXPRESS
ANGER

"Cancer sucks, plain and simple. But what it brings with it is so complex. Cancer has taken so much from me but also brought so much good into my life. I have had the opportunity to meet so many amazing people and have been so inspired to love everyday because you just are not promised tomorrow. If we are lucky enough to have tomorrow, make it matter. Be kind, be patient. be true, breathe and laugh. People may not always remember exactly what you say but they will remember how you make them feel.

The power of connection is magical and I am grateful to have had this fantastic experience. Thank you all so much!"

—JACKIE HERIGODT, INSPIRATION

"From the first minutes we met virtually on Zoom, it felt like we've been friends for years. I'm so grateful to Jackie for taking the time to share her story and collaborate with me on this piece. I am in complete awe of her continuous work to help those affected by cancer in her role at Imerman Angels, so it's an honor to be given the opportunity to help her share her own story. We took all the words she associated with cancer—anything and everything—and integrated them into the artwork. In the end, we created a beautiful juxtaposition of light and dark on the canvas together.

This is Jackie's story, but a familiar story to so many others. Our hope is that this serves as a reminder that we will always carry around some bits of darkness, but it's the light and love in our lives that help us continue to heal and stay looking forward."

—JEFF GUERRERO, ARTIST

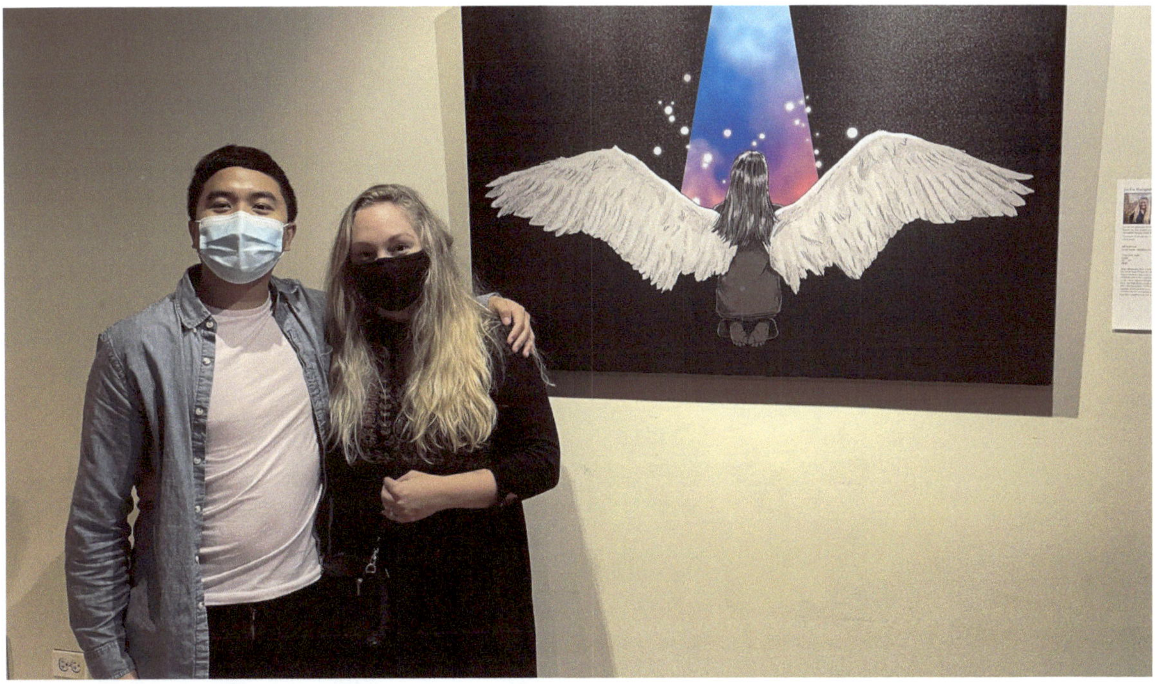

JEFF & JACKIE AT THE BWC MIDWEST GALA

heal

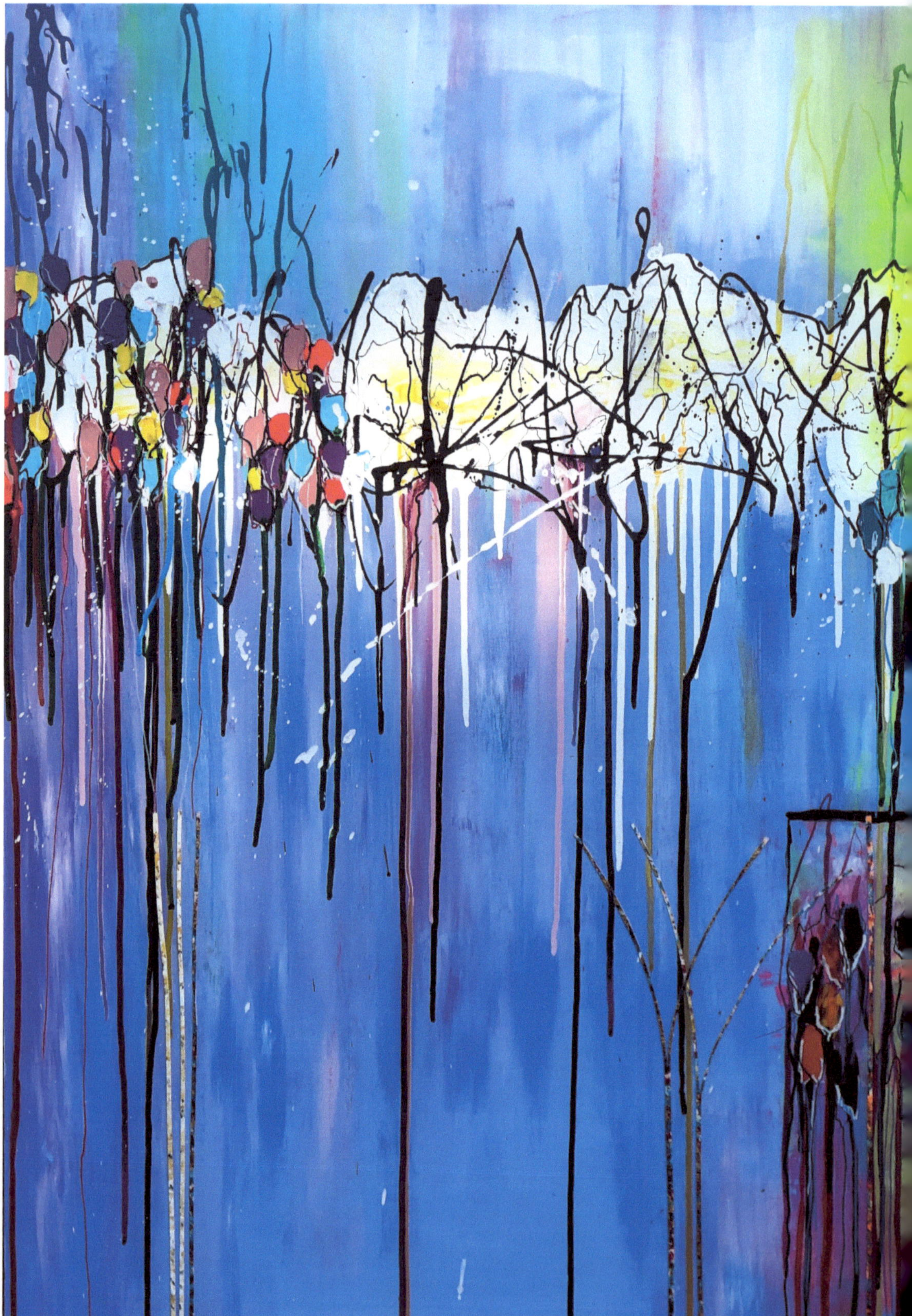

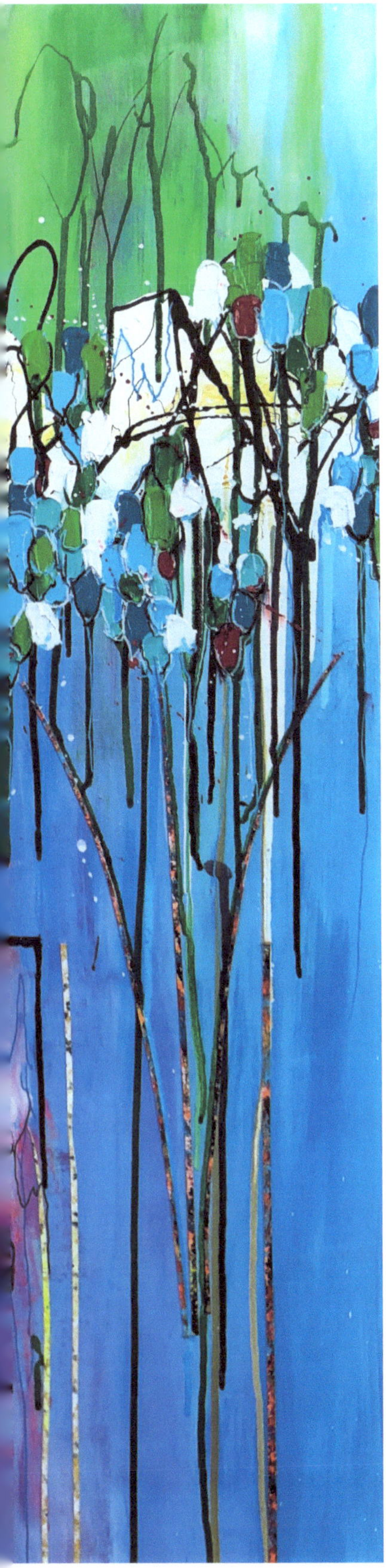

"Tulips"

Inspiration: Mardi Kaplan
Artist: Anna Feneis

BWC Chicago, 2020

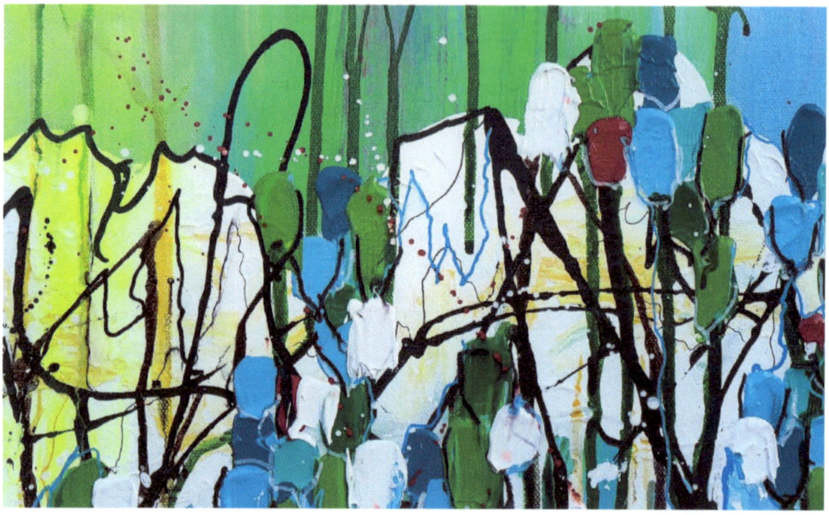

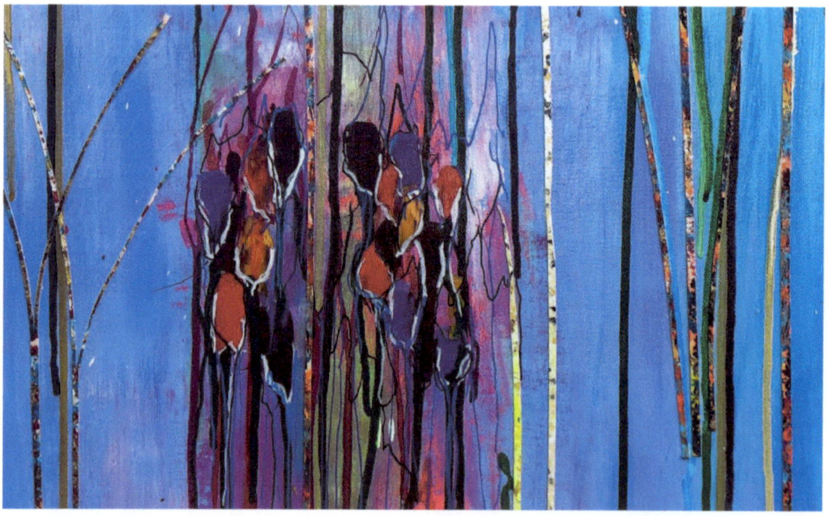

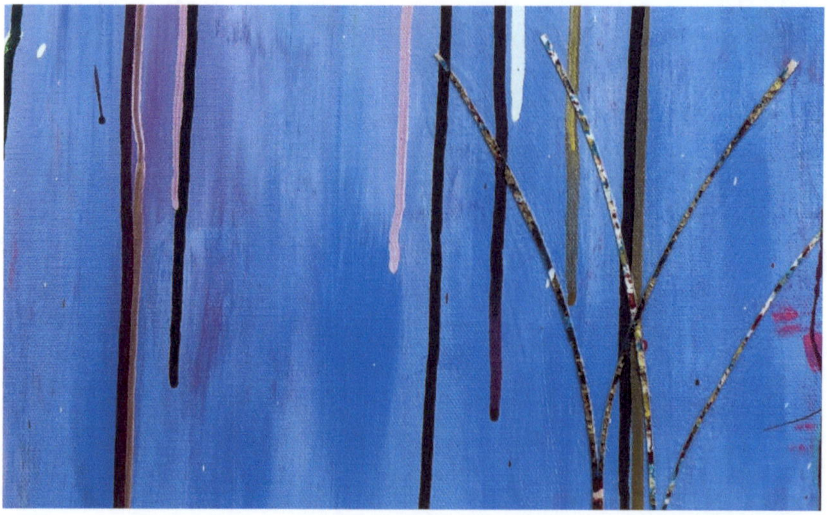

A Surprising Connection

Anna Feneis had participated as a Brushes with Cancer Chicago Artist prior to being paired with Inspiration Mardi Kaplan, but nothing could prepare her for her 2020 experience with Kaplan.

"Every time I hung up with Mardi, I felt like I could have talked for two more hours," Feneis said. "I would look at my husband and say 'I have never felt so safe and natural right off the bat.'"

Shortly after the two connected, Feneis' father, also an artist, was diagnosed with cancer. If that wasn't difficult enough to come to terms with, a dear friend was diagnosed for a third time. Feneis was luckily in the right company.

"I don't know why they paired us, but there was some sort of hand in it," Feneis said. "Talking to Mardi and learning her story was therapy for me because I could come to her. It was really lucky."

Feneis was particularly inspired by the way Kaplan handled her breast cancer diagnosis, treatment and recovery. A week after Kaplan was diagnosed with breast cancer, she left for Morocco.
"I look back and think, maybe I did that knowing I wouldn't be going anywhere for a while," Kaplan said.

That's how Kaplan set the tone for her cancer journey: she wasn't going to let it get in the way of the things that brought her joy. By continuing on with life, Kaplan had an opportunity to face her diagnosis head on.

"She went on a trip to Morocco right after

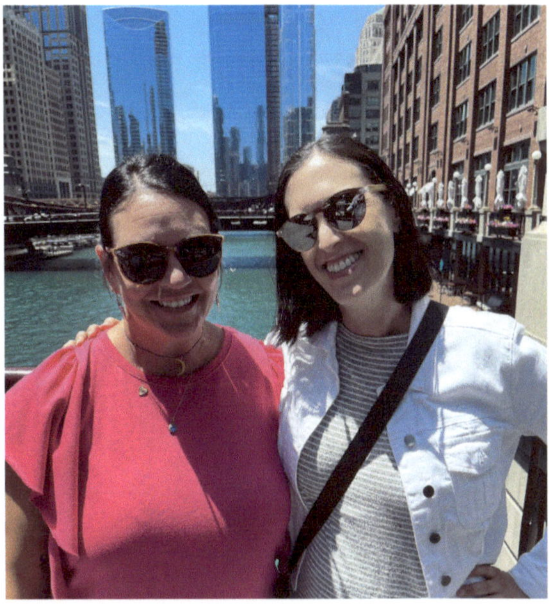

ANNA FENEIS & MARDI KAPLAN

getting diagnosed!" Feneis said. "That's what I want my kids to do. I want my daughters to hear something that scares them, do their research, learn about it and move forward."

The two built such a connection they decided to merge both their cancer journeys into one. Feneis took a painting of her father's, cut it up and used the strips as ferns in her Brushes with Cancer piece for Kaplan.

"I feel like this was such a two-sided experience," Kaplan said. "Even the piece of art isn't about me, it's about our relationship – all the colors and craziness of it."

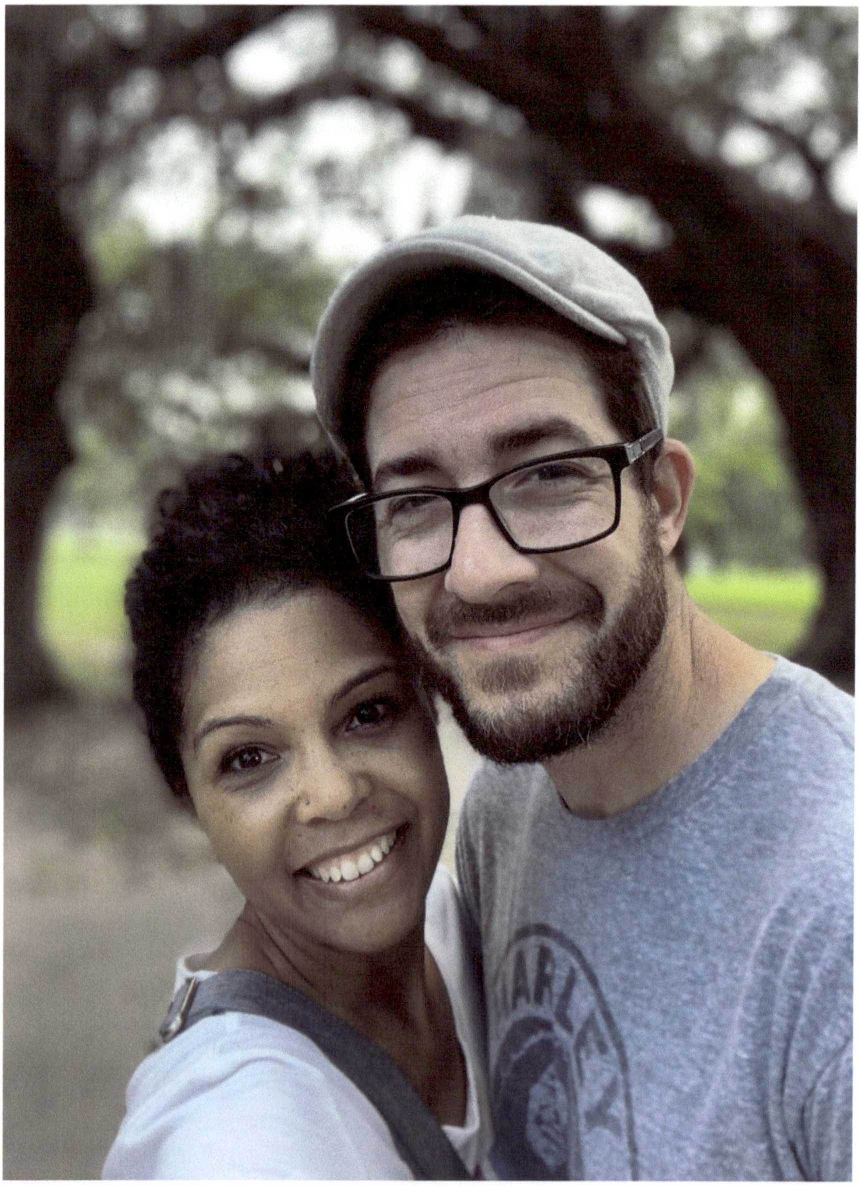

AUGUST SPREE & BRAD YOUNG

A Twist Love Story

WRITTEN BY AUGUST SPREE

It was a breezy April evening, and I happened to get a ticket from a co-worker to an event called "Brushes with Cancer" that started right after work. Without having any idea what to expect, I walked the six blocks or so to the event. It had been 10 years since my first cancer diagnosis and only a couple months since a recurrence scare. In addition to being a cancer survivor myself, my grandmother was diagnosed with stomach cancer a few years after my experience, and she passed away only 10 months later. I was eager to be connected within the cancer community.

As I observed the event throughout the evening, my heart was touched and I remember thinking, "What is this? This artwork is so amazing. How did they do all this?" as I walked around the venue reading the stories next to each work of art. I asked one of the artists who was responsible for all this and he pointed me in the direction of Jenna. When I found a moment to introduce myself to her, I jokingly said, "My name is August, I am a cancer survivor, and we are going to be friends!" and she very graciously laughed and agreed to have coffee with me soon.

Over the next two years, I told everyone I knew about Twist Out Cancer. I began recruiting my closest friends, family and even acquaintances to be involved with the Brushes with Cancer program. And then, one day after a phone call, Jenna suggested I participate as an Inspiration in the 2014 Brushes program.

With my artist Brad Young, I could talk about how I thought I was going to faint when the doctor told me the biopsy results, how I felt my baby kicking in my belly while I struggled to make my way back to my car after that appointment (I was eight months pregnant at the time of diagnosis), how I felt guilty that I didn't have the strength to call my best friend and tell her so I sent her an email instead, and so many other things. I was able to lay out all of my journey, the fears, the struggles, and the victories, without judgment, criticism or emotional reaction. And while I shared, I could feel myself coming to terms with my own experiences.

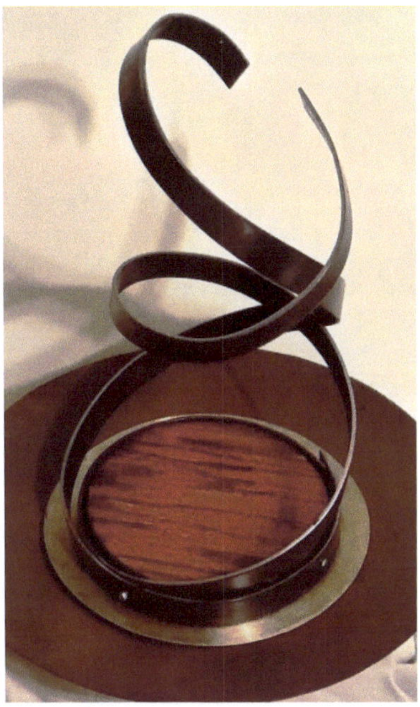

"The Dance"

Inspiration: August Spree
Artist: Brad Young

BWC Chicago, 2014

Since that initial experience in Brushes with Cancer, my artist and I have become partners in many ways and we now live together in Chicago. That first night when I walked into the Brushes with Cancer event, I knew my life had changed but I had no way of knowing just how much. From growth and healing through the Brushes program, to the expansion of my heart and new love, to becoming an Executive Board Member and ambassador of Twist Out Cancer and the Brushes with Cancer program, my life has been altered in the best possible ways because of this experience.

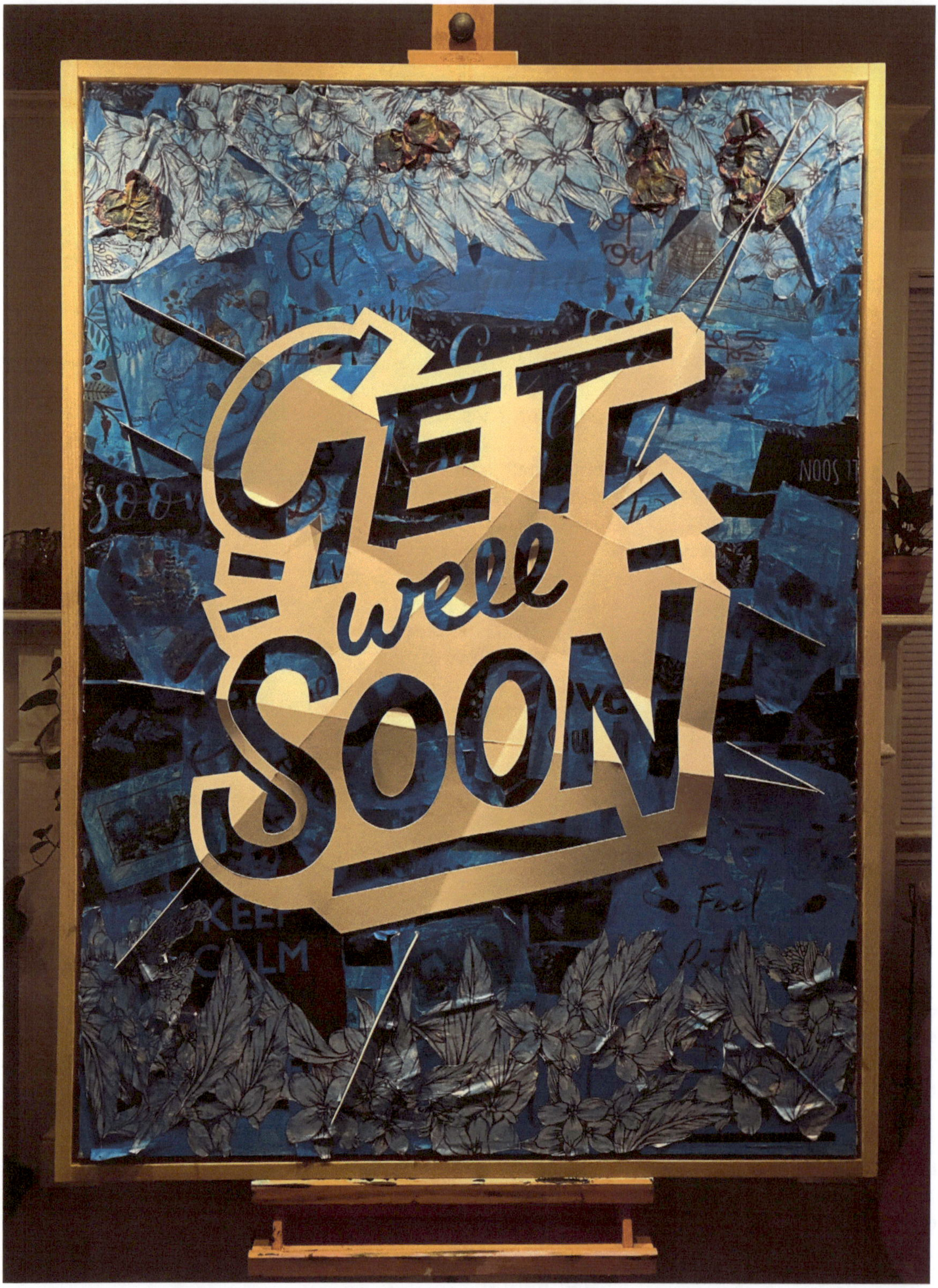

"Platitudes: Blue Ocean of Emotion"

Inspiration: Kathleen Brown
Artist: John Stumbaugh

Platitudes in the Spotlight

While Kathleen Brown was going through her cancer journey, she was completely overwhelmed by get-well cards. They came in droves and collected in Hefty bags. There were so many that some were never opened.

Brown was 13 and a week away from beginning eighth grade when she was diagnosed with Ewing's sarcoma, a rare form of bone cancer. Her treatment took 15 months.

"I was a very avid athlete at the time and had no symptoms outside exercise-induced asthma," Brown said. "Within three months of diagnosis, I was given my last rights and blessed by Joseph Cardinal Bernardin, the late Archbishop of the Chicago Catholic Church.

After 15 months of grueling treatment, she finished on Dec. 2, 1996. It took nearly 15 years for Brown to begin emotionally healing from the experience.

"Treatment was hard on all of us, but recovery was so much harder," Brown said. "In those days nobody was talking about mental health or providing support. It was all focused on getting to the end of treatment."

It wasn't until 2010 that she sought mental health support to sort through the complex emotions.

"You get to the end and you are like, 'What now? How do I return to whatever normal life is and how do I deal with these emotions?' When you're in fight-or-flight mode, it's a race to the finish line."

Artist John Stumbaugh was ready to tackle some of those complex emotions alongside Brown. No stranger to Twist Out Cancer and the Brushes with Cancer programs, Stumbaugh's whole family is part of the TOC community. This year was Stumbaugh's third as a Brushes with Cancer Artist and his wife and daughter have both participated in the program.

As they got to know each other, Stumbaugh learned about the card-filled Hefty bags and Brown's feelings toward empty platitudes.

"Becoming aware of platitudes, especially now, has been important," he said. "People are giving well wishes in the best way they know how, but it's overwhelming for the person."

"Platitudes" are like pick-me-up clichés. You've heard them so many times they've become empty. "Get well soon," "Every cloud has a silver lining," "Everything happens for a reason." While well intentioned, these sentiments can often do harm to those receiving them.

Stumbaugh knew this had to be the focus of the piece, and that Brown had to be involved in the process.

"Early on, I went to Walgreens, bought greeting cards and started tearing the cards apart," he said. "That was the start of the process: let's tear things up. I don't know what that will look like, but let's put this on a canvas."

The duo searched for cards on a free website to print off and tear up. Being in the middle of COVID-19, they took turns tearing up the cards – working together but apart.

"Something was powerful for me in that learning process," Stumbaugh said. "The idea of tearing it up was powerful and unexpected in a good way."

Having Brown involved only furthered her healing.

"This process is a great way to express yourself and feelings that come up in cancer treatment and also in isolation," she said.

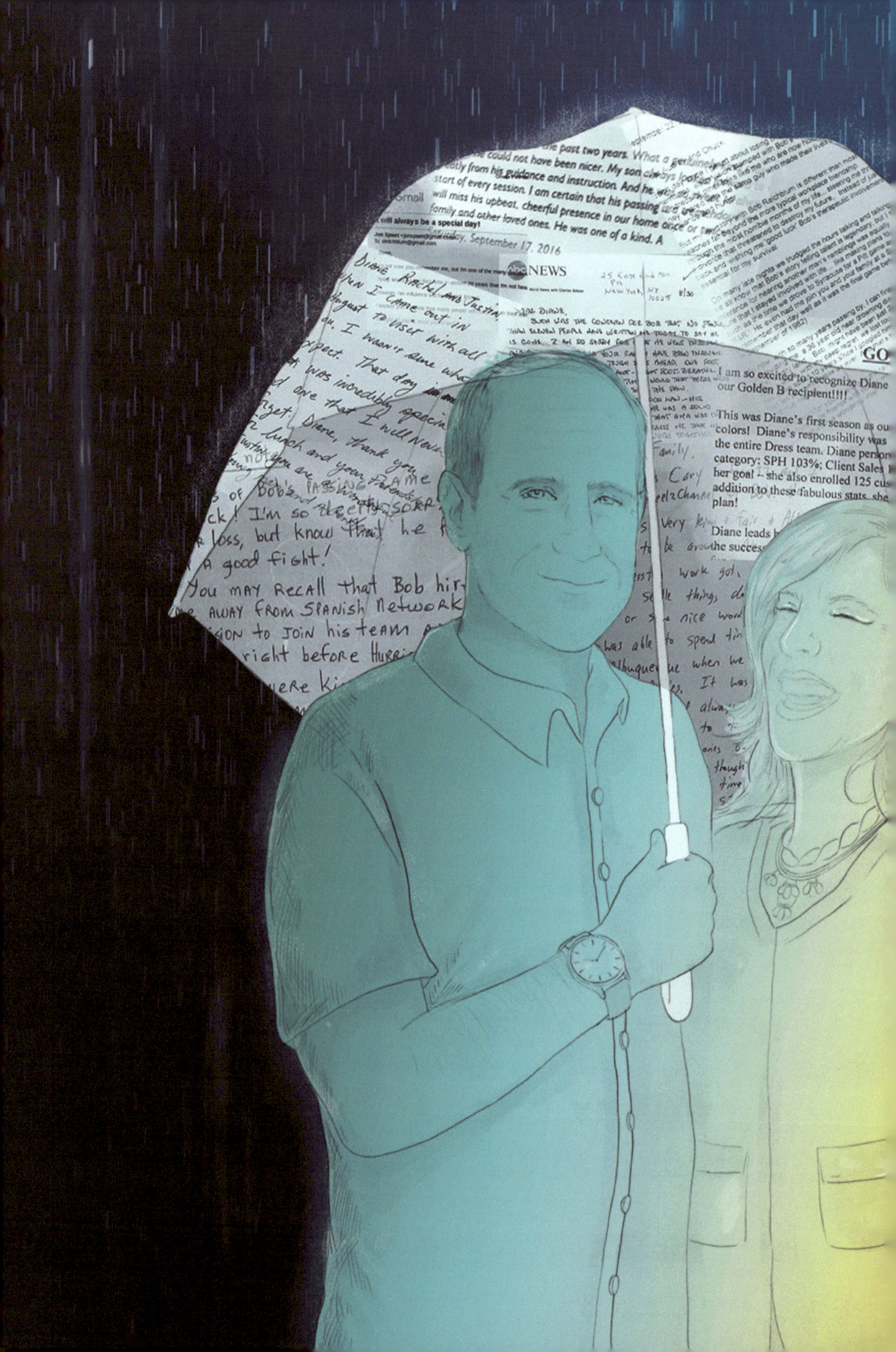

the past two years. What a gem
could not have been nicer. My son
atly from his guidance and instruction. And he
start of every session. I am certain that his passing
will miss his upbeat, cheerful presence in our home once
family and other loved ones. He was one of a kind. A
will always be a special day!
September 17, 2016
NEWS
Diane, Rachel and Justin,
When I came out in
August to visit with all
expect. That day
was incredibly special
and one that I will never
forget. Diane, thank you
lunch and your friendship
you are
of Bob's passing. So sorry
ck! I'm so
loss, but know that he f
a good fight!
You may recall that Bob hir
away from Spanish Network
to join his team
right before Hurri
were ki
I am so excited to recognize Diane
our Golden B recipient!!!!
This was Diane's first season as ou
colors! Diane's responsibility was
the entire Dress team. Diane person
category: SPH 103%; Client Sales
her goal – she also enrolled 125 cus
addition to these fabulous stats, she
plan!
Diane leads b
the success

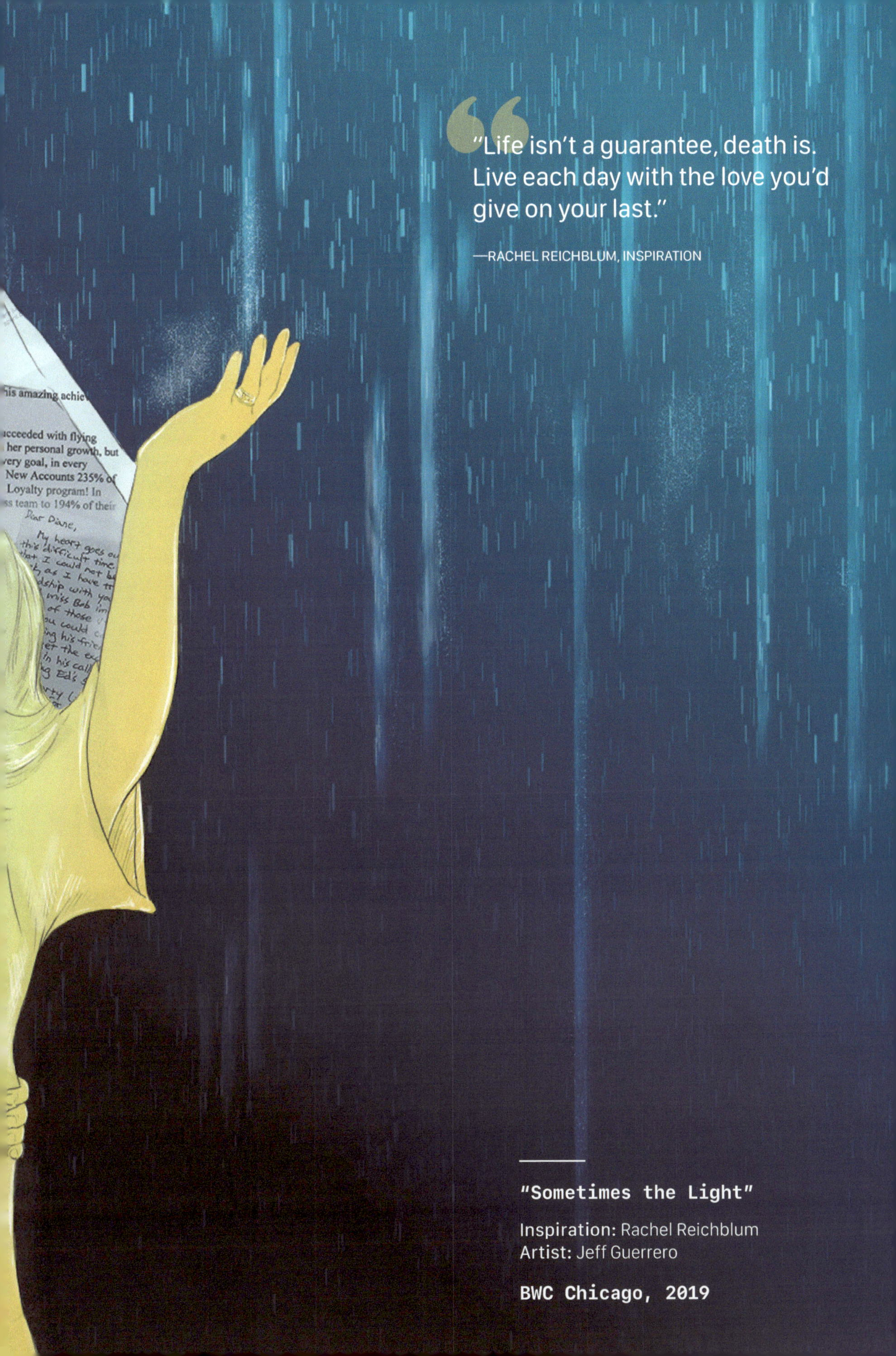

"Life isn't a guarantee, death is. Live each day with the love you'd give on your last."

—RACHEL REICHBLUM, INSPIRATION

"Sometimes the Light"

Inspiration: Rachel Reichblum
Artist: Jeff Guerrero

BWC Chicago, 2019

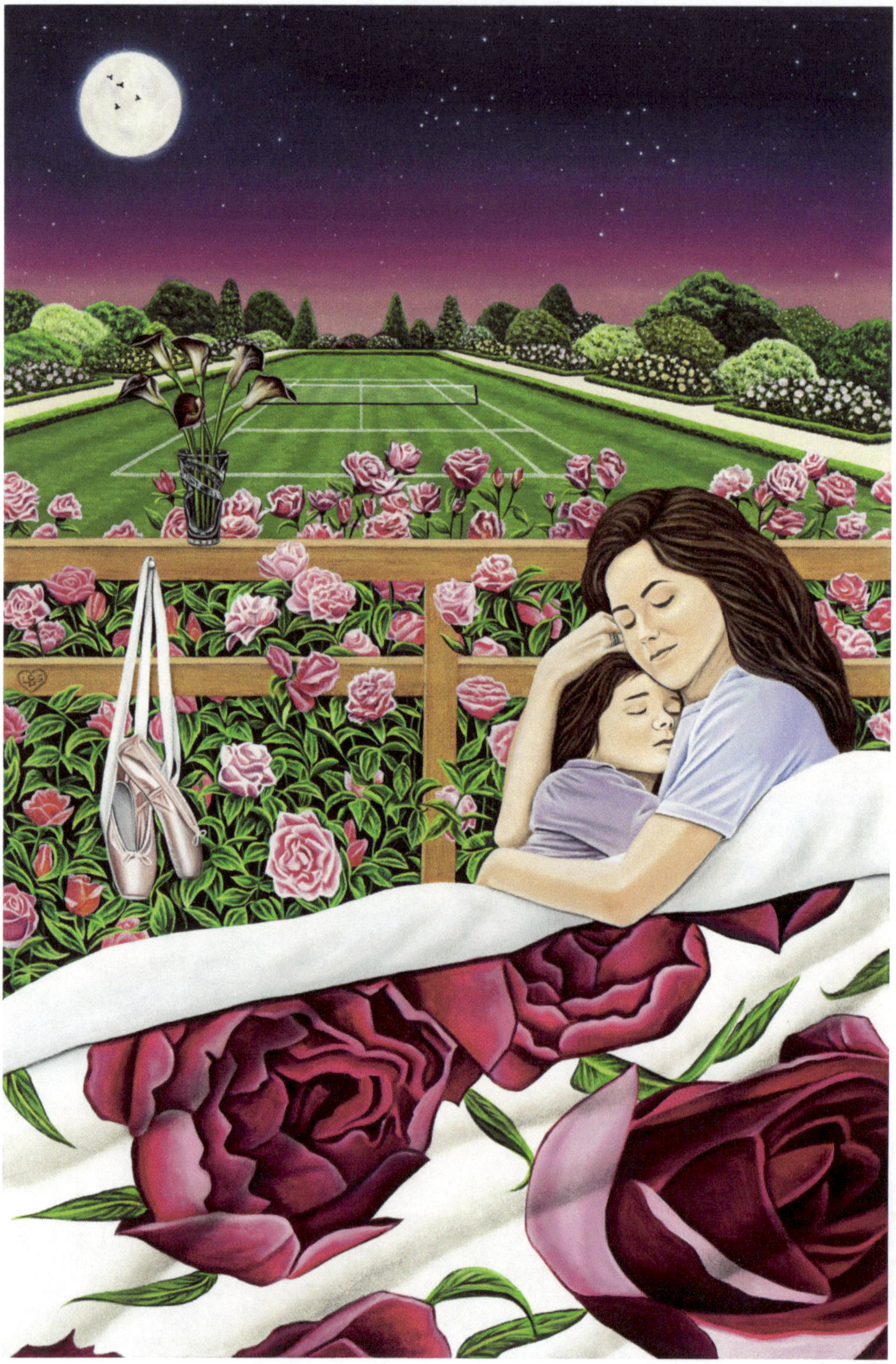

"Embrace"

Inspiration: Lisa Glick
Artist: Nicole Gordon

BWC Chicago, 2020

A Mother's Love

Coming up on nine years since her mother Lois' passing, Lisa Glick was invited to take part in Brushes with Cancer as an Inspiration. She had attended the previous year's event in Chicago and was deeply touched by the featured Artists and Inspirations. Honored by the extended invite, she accepted and was paired with Artist Nicole Gordon.

The Glick family has long been an important part of the Twist Out Cancer community, with Lisa's brother Danny serving as a generous donor and the Chicago 2020 Event Honoree. Now, it was time to honor Lisa, who served as Lois' caregiver for 13 months.

When it became clear that Lois' condition was terminal, Lisa began reaching out to family and friends near and far who had touched and or had been touched by Lois' life with the message: "If you have to make a choice between visiting Lois while she is living or attending her funeral, you should visit Lois WHILE SHE IS LIVING."

Lisa and Lois found joy and humor in some of the most unusual circumstances. Routine tasks, like bathing, toileting and dressing often required creativity which ultimately led to hysterical laughter.

"Caring for my mother was the most joyful and intimate experience of my life. I knew every inch of her body, her thoughts and how to care for her. It was an amazing journey," Lisa said.

She remembers one particularly poignant moment when she and Lois were at a follow-up appointment with Lois's surgical oncologist.

"As we waited for the doctor, we looked deep into each other's eyes lovingly and intensely," Lisa said. Then, my mother said 'I gave you your life, now you are giving me mine.' It was at this moment our roles changed. I would become her lifeline until her passing."

When Lisa connected with her Artist Nicole, it was the duo's instant connection that fueled Nicole's creativity. Their natural chemistry made it less like a project with a due date and more like friends getting to know one another better.

"It didn't feel like I was carrying the story of a stranger, it was really interesting," Nicole said. "As Lisa was speaking and telling me her stories, every once in a while, she would reveal a story that immediately clicked as a visual image."

Nicole would "collect" these stories as images for her piece. It was important that she connect the work to Lisa whenever possible.

"In this piece, there are details hidden everywhere that are symbols," Nicole said. "I wanted the whole painting to be filled with little pieces of Lisa. Learning about Lisa's story is so moving. As a recipient of the storytelling, it was really powerful."

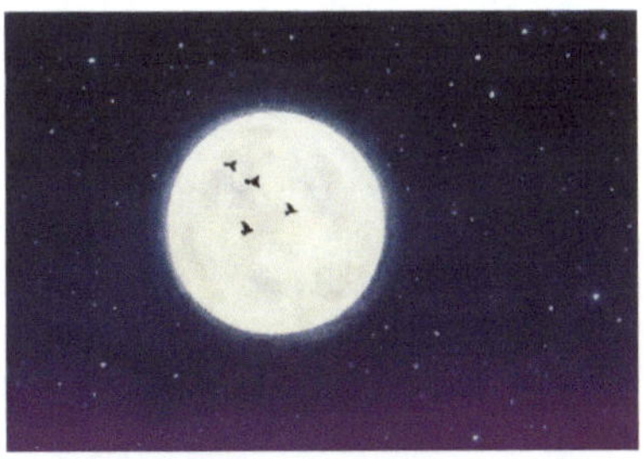

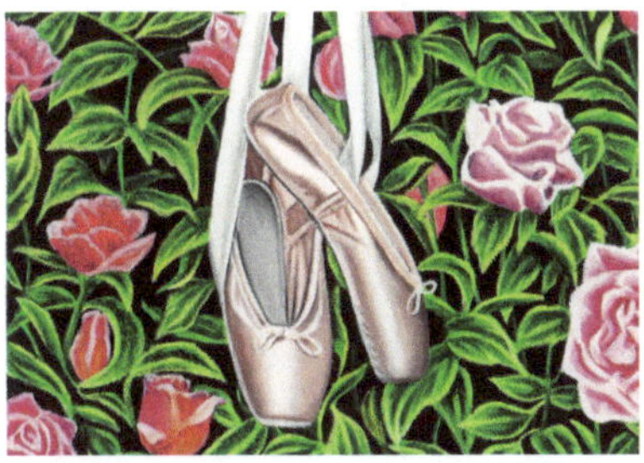

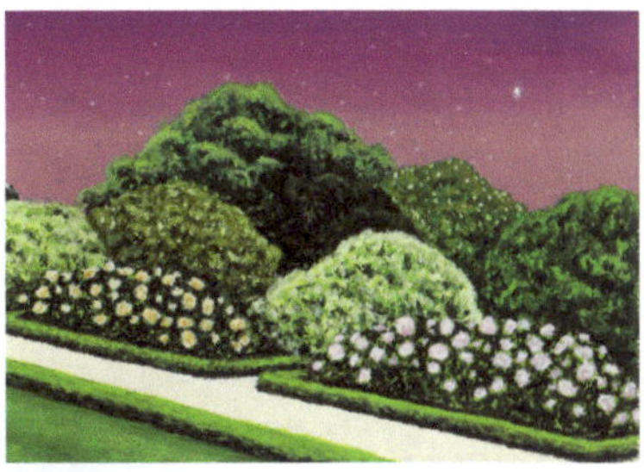

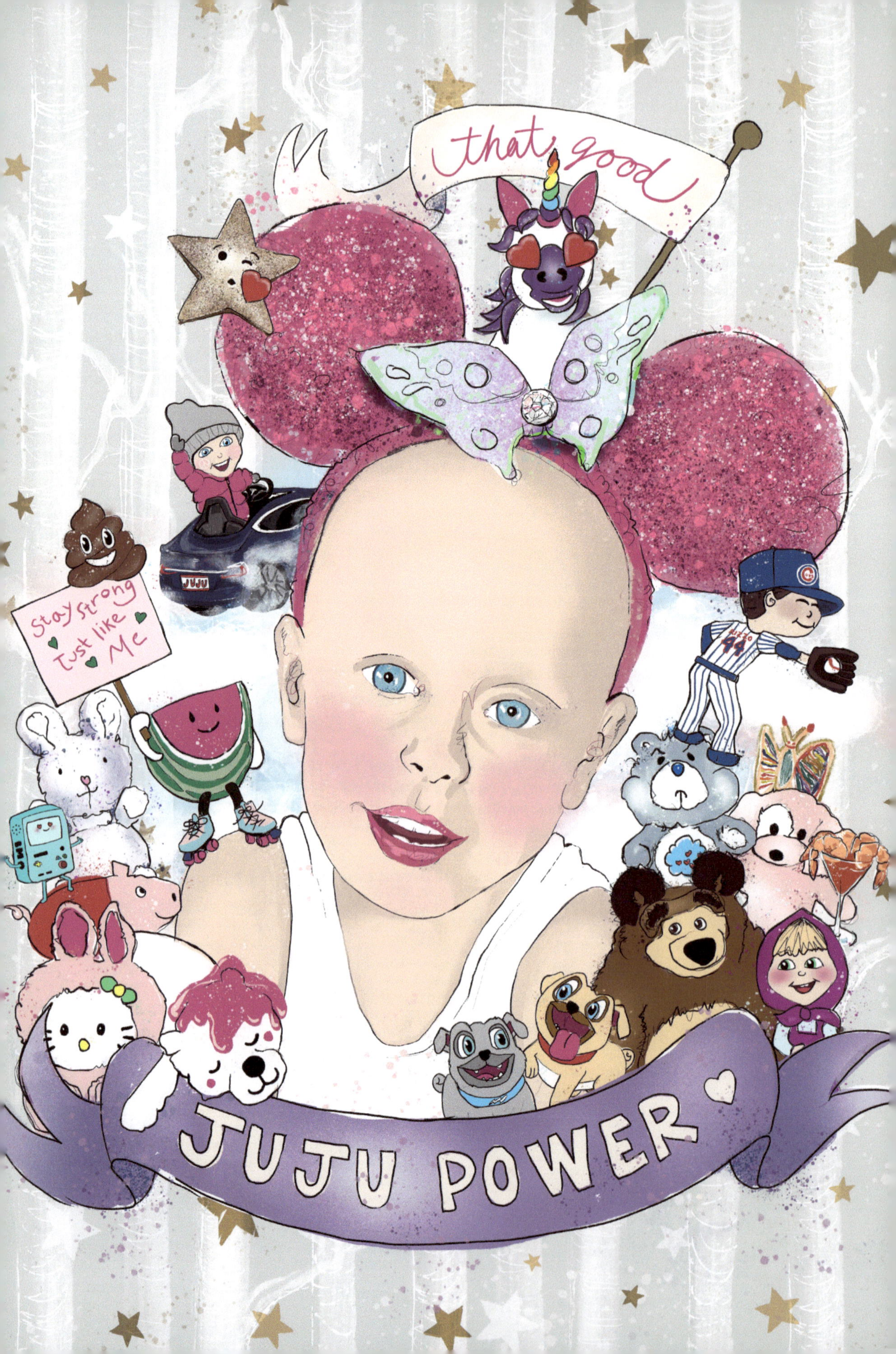
that good
Stay strong
Just like Me
JUJU POWER

"My brush with cancer was as a caregiver for my 5-year old daughter, Juliana, during her very courageous battle with Neuroblastoma. Yes, I certainly learned that pediatric cancer deserves more attention and funding. Yes, I saw firsthand how pediatric hospitals fill these children's hospital stays with so much love and hope and the oncology nurses and doctors are true modern-day superheroes. But the thing that perhaps was most noticeable was how each and every child we met battling cancer was truly a warrior. Each one was so special, brave and resilient. It was somewhat surreal; like they were handpicked to confront this horrendous disease because they were the only ones who stood the chance to overcome it. So many people were inspired by Juliana's battle that 'JuJu Power' quickly came about. It represented JuJu's ability to confront such a difficult obstacle in a super human, awe-inspiring manner.

We are incredibly grateful to Brushes with Cancer and especially Melissa Burgess who immediately understood JuJu's vibrant, colorful and heroic nature through her beautiful piece of artwork."

—STACI GREENFIELD, INSPIRATION

"When I met my Inspiration, Staci, I was so touched by her brush with cancer. She spoke about her amazing daughter Juliana, or JuJu for short, and how, in Juju's brief 5 years on this earth, she brought out laughter, love and wonder in every person she met. Staci called it her 'JuJu Power,' and as I learned more, I felt that power too.

I'm a professional photographer by trade, but when Staci showed me around JuJu's magical bedroom filled with so many of the things that made her happy, my imagination kicked in and I immediately thought of this squishy, colorful world where JuJu and her favorite things could exist and play together - I could just see her bringing her stuffed toys and cartoons to life around her, and I knew this was the perfect chance for me to jump into an illustrated portrait instead.

While the many playful references in this piece are inside nods to her family and best friends, I worked to showcase That Good JuJu Power in a way that could pull you into her imaginary world, and make you want to experience it too!"

—MELISSA BURGESS, ARTIST

"That Good JuJu Power"

Inspiration: Staci Greenfield
Artist: Melissa Burgess

BWC Chicago, 2020

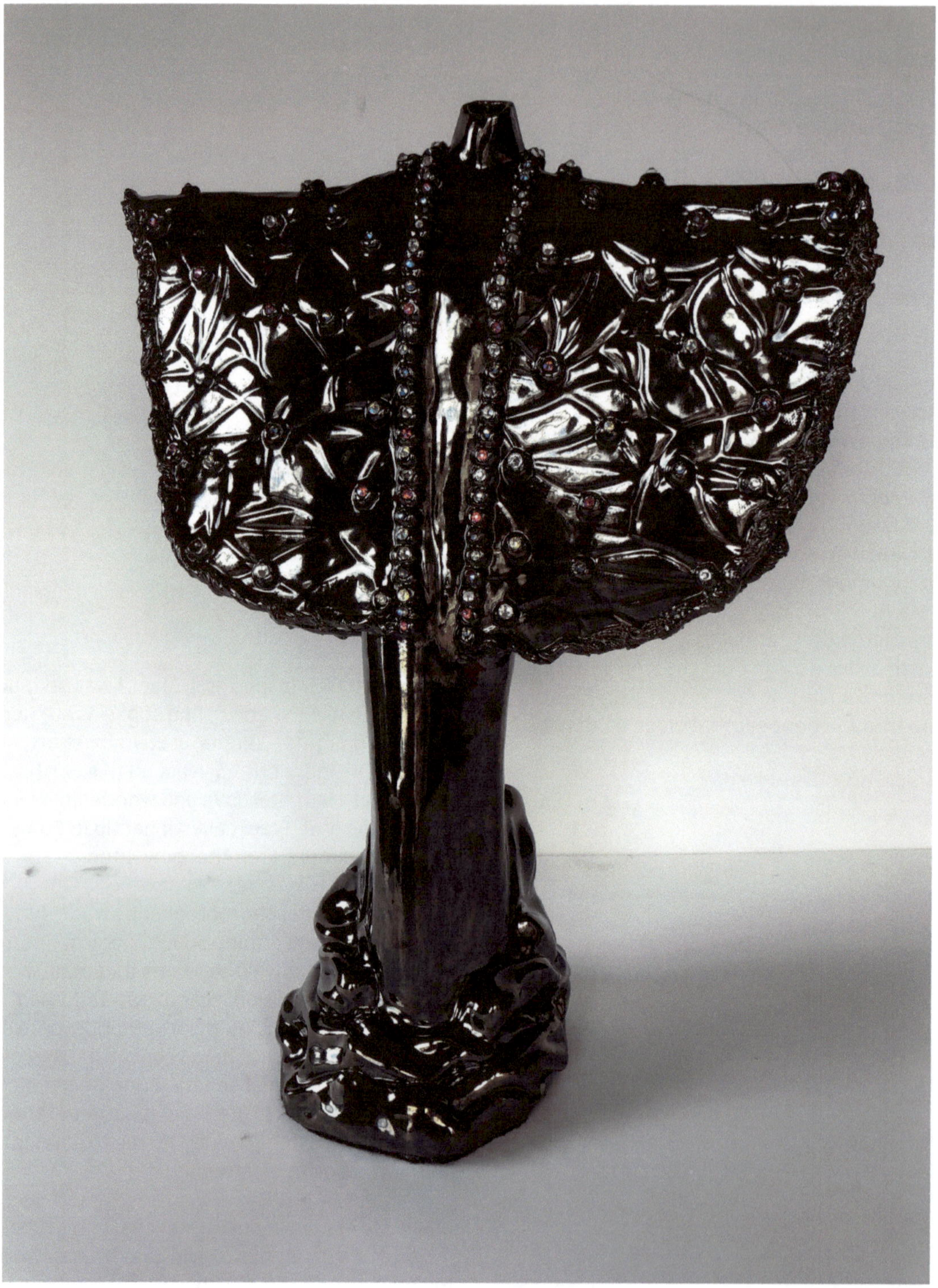

"Open Circuit"

Inspiration: Roger Joseph Mommaerts, Jr.
Artist: Renee Chase

BWC Austin, 2020

"Cancer is hard... sometimes it leaves you disfigured and/or disabled, but I keep fighting. Cancer has taught me to not give up, to continue living life. Don't stop! Share your cancer experience so that others may learn and become more aware."

—ROGER JOSEPH MOMMAERTS, JR., INSPIRATION

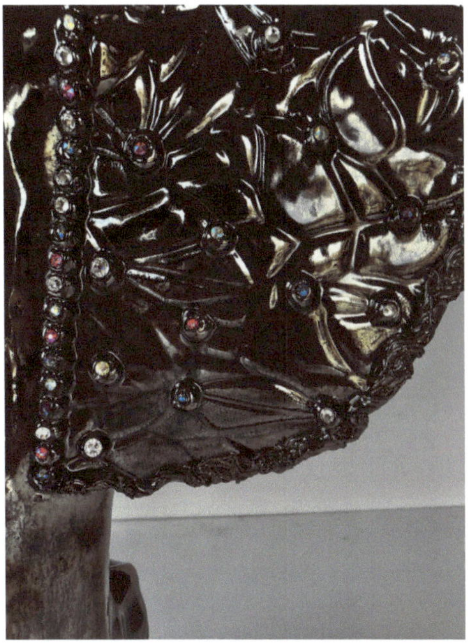

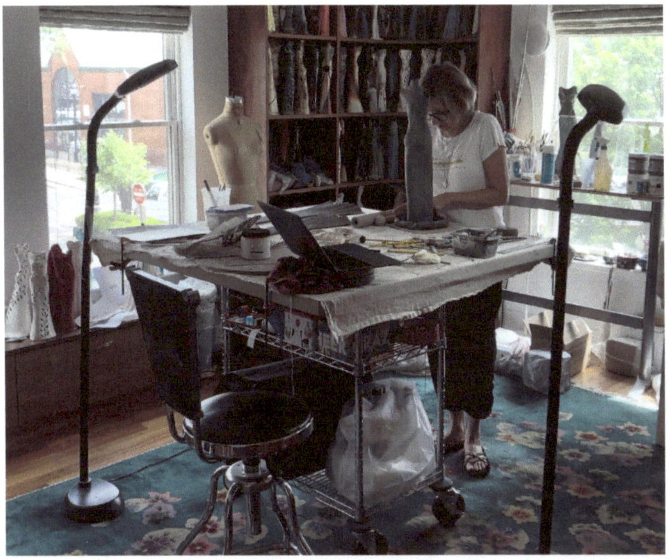

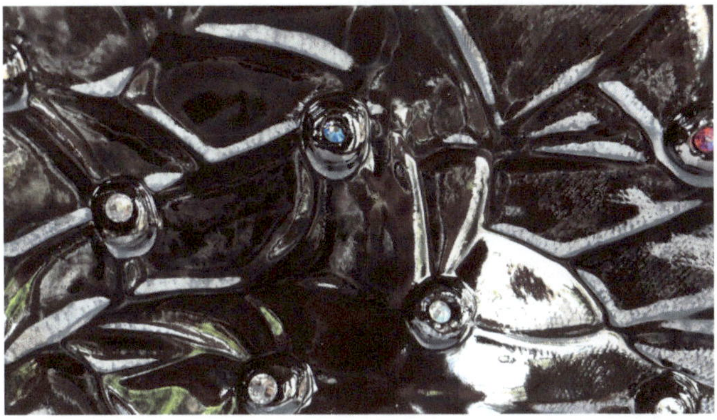

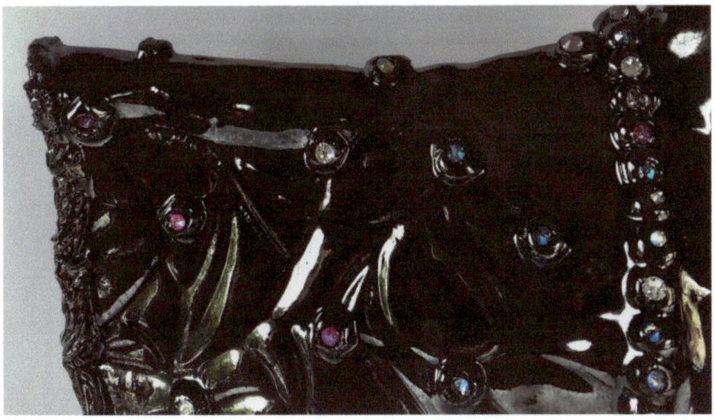

"My inspiration is a lovely man, Roger, who has been battling brain cancer for a great part of his life. After hearing about his ongoing journey, I was concerned about how a designer/dressmaker/sculptor who focused on the female form would relay Roger's strength and hope. Through my conversation with him, I learned that what carries him through the profound challenge in his life is his wife, Holly. My focus then became clear.

The brain is the basis of all we do and all we are able to do, so I started with that imagery as the foundation for my piece. From the cerebrum and cerebellum grew the angel. With outspread wings of hope, dark and reflective, she protects and embraces. Her cape-wings are covered with the patterns of neurons, the axons and dendrites colliding and intersecting; each point marked by the light of a Swarovski crystal.

Although the sculpture is a hollow form without indication of body parts, I strived to fill it with emotion so that the viewer could imagine the soul that lives within."

—RENEE CHASE, ARTIST

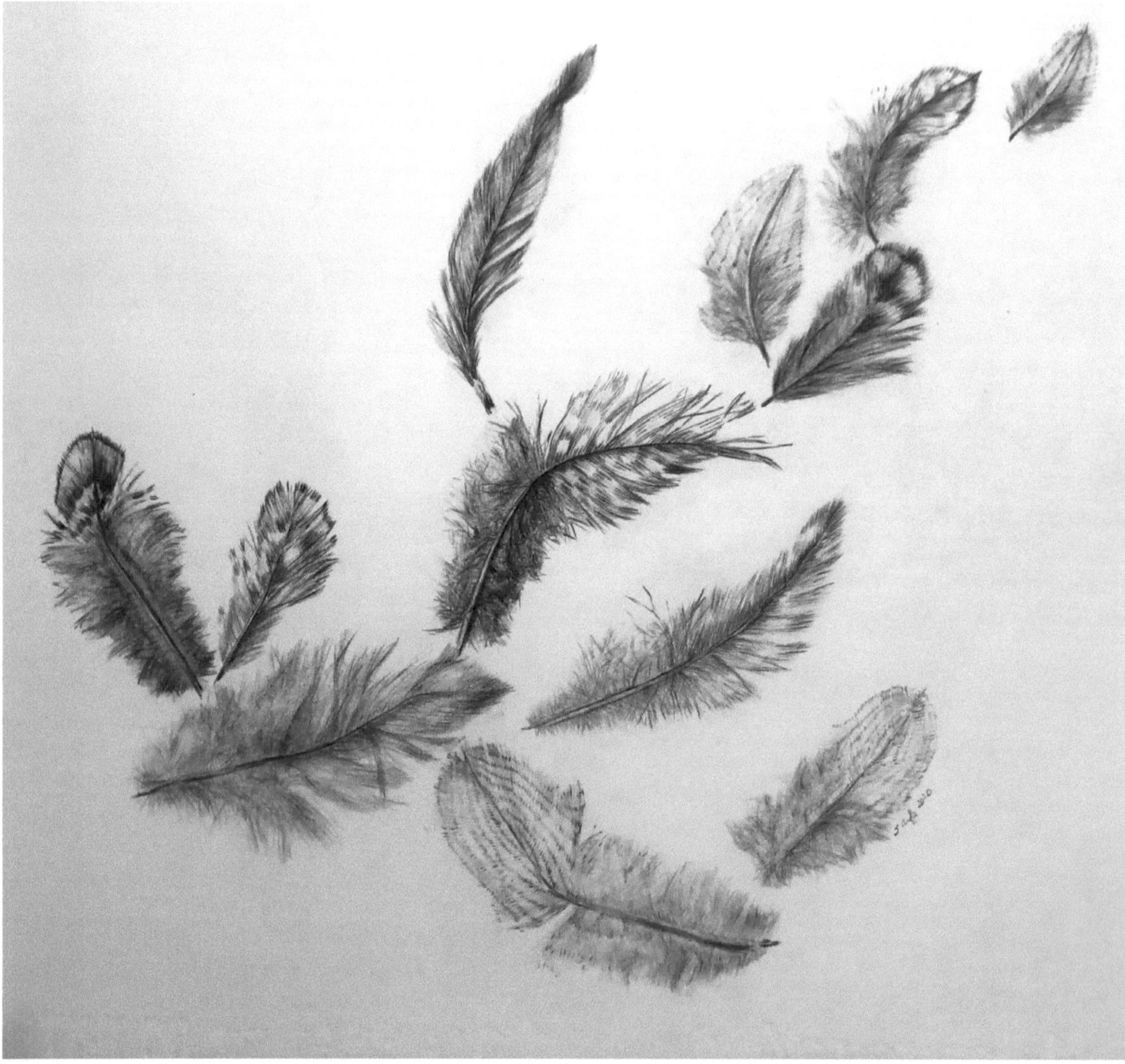

"Uplifted"

Inspiration: Raychel Funk
Artist: Dr. Sharon Arffa

BWC Austin, 2020

How Dr. Sharon Arffa Finds Healing as a Brushes with Cancer Artist

When Dr. Sharon Arffa learned about Twist Out Cancer, she knew she had to be part of its Brushes with Cancer program. Her psychology world and her art world were finally about to collide.

"Brushes with Cancer is remarkable, for me as a healer, to heal in a very different way – it was just eye opening," she said. "I think, as an artist, depicting something extremely meaningful in an art form is much more amazing than just creating something pretty."

Since her experience as a Brushes with Cancer Artist, Arffa has been an active part of the Twist Out Cancer community, with her involvement ranging from generous donations to serving on the TOC Executive Board.

"There has not been as an intense or rewarding experience as Brushes with Cancer," she said. "I'm not sure I can explain it."

Arffa was prepared to be an empathetic ear when she was paired with her 2018 Brushes with Cancer Inspiration, Raychel. While Arffa has not been touched by cancer personally, her brother is currently having his own cancer journey that understandably affects the entire family.

She also has a deep understanding of what it's like to pick yourself up after severe trauma. Shortly after Arffa and her husband celebrated their 35th anniversary, he tragically passed away in a plane crash. The next few years were filled with pain for the Arffa family, however, human connection is what helped get them through the unthinkable.

"It's wonderful there are people out there who help you," she said. "I had such a response from my friends - that was a wonderful experience."

For Brushes with Cancer, Arffa was able to pull from her own personal experiences, as well as her training as a psychologist and artist. As a healer, Arffa says seeing a new way to heal through the Brushes with Cancer experience offered her personal growth in a unique way.

"There was part of me that got better – it wasn't necessarily healing my previous trauma, instead I was able to connect in such an amazing manner with someone."

The experience prompted her to get even more involved in Twist Out Cancer, becoming integral to the community.

"Part of me feels the need to give back to others and not let other people suffer. You always suffer with some of this but there are ways to ease that."

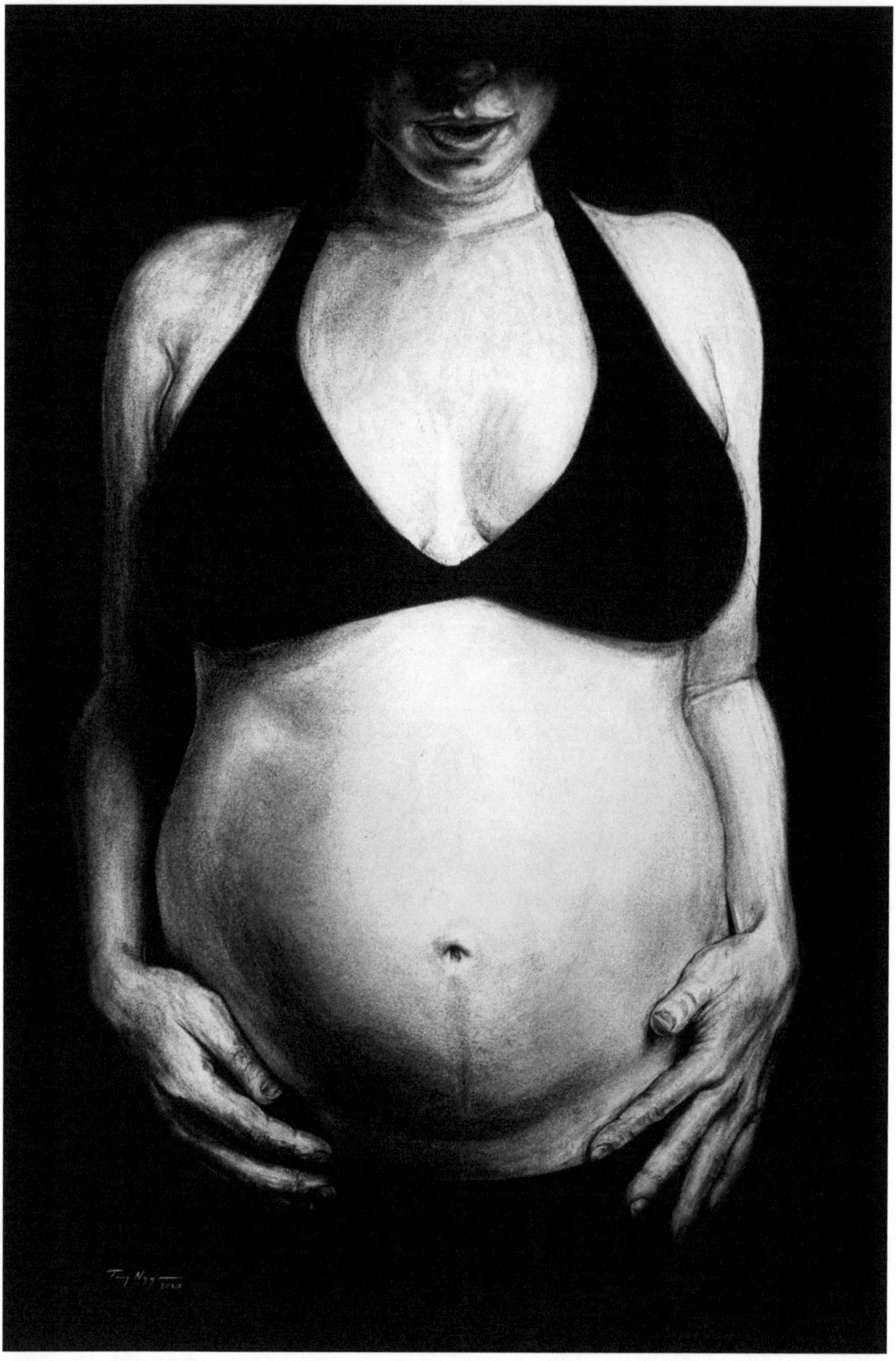

"Motherhood"

Inspiration: Fayruz Benyousef
Artist: Tony Nguyen

A Family Begins to Heal After Multiple Cancer Journeys

To understand Fayruz Benyousef's cancer journey, you have to go back to 1980.

Benyousef was living with her family in Pennsylvania when her dad was diagnosed with acute leukemia. Both her mother, Dr. Nuria Treki, and father, Sharif Benyousef, had no history of cancer. For the Libyan family, the diagnosis was devastating.

"Culturally, getting cancer was a death sentence," Benyousef said.

After extreme challenges with his chemo treatment, Sharif went into remission and began a job as a civil engineer. But eight years later, the family was devastated once more.

"I went to take a shower and saw swelling on my collar bone," Benyousef said. "It didn't hurt and I didn't feel bad, but I showed it to my mom and she went white."

After going through a painful cycle with cancer, the family was hit again. Benyousef had stage 2B Hodgkin's Lymphoma. While Benyousef worked to pick up the pieces after exhausting treatment during the summer before her junior year of high school, Sharif relapsed. The Leukemia came back and it was much more aggressive. About six weeks into her senior year of high school, Benyousef got the call to drop everything and fly to Pittsburgh so she could say goodbye to her father. Tragically, she did not make it in time.

"I thought I'd get to say goodbye, but there was a miscommunication," she said. "Instead, I walked into a dead body. I was talking to him and touching his feet, and when the nurse walked by, I asked why the monitor wasn't there."

More than 20 years later, the two were thrust back into the unthinkable. Memorial weekend 2018 was just underway and when Benyousef and her mother went to urgent care, they immediately sent them to the hospital. Dr. Treki had stage 4 metastatic breast cancer.

"She probably has known for 10 years that something was not right," Benyousef said. "But because of her fear and trauma from my father's experience, she did not want to go to the doctor."

Benyousef focused on caring for her mother, as well as a successful career, loving marriage and beautiful child. One day, she noticed she had chest pain accompanied by a hardness. She thought it was a cyst, but her husband encouraged her to get it checked immediately. Cancer was back – six months after her mother was diagnosed.

Through Twist Out Cancer and the power of the arts, Beyousef and Dr. Treki are focusing on beautiful memories to help heal the difficult ones.

"This experience is reigniting those passions and bringing a joy we'd never have without Twist Out Cancer," Benyousef said. "It's so heartwarming and a way to help heal by bringing back things that are happy memories, like being with dad."

Dr. Treki – an accomplished singer – was paired with artist Kenzie Slottow, a flutist who asked Beyousef and Dr. Treki to sing in the piece. The three have had a few Zoom meetings with her and both Beyousef and her mother are enjoying reconnecting with their passion for music.

"That's been part of the joy – reconnecting with the past," Beyousef said. "I grew up in a house where music was always playing – mom and dad were always singing together. It was a beautifully romantic era. It was a happy life and music and art were core and central to it."

"Cancer was a sucker punch to the gut when I was diagnosed. It's been a scary journey that I never would have chosen to go on. Cancer has also done a great deal of good. It's given me confidence, an appreciation for who I am and the life I have and I will never take myself, the life that I'm living or the people in my life for granted again. I am a wife. I am a mom. I am a daughter and granddaughter. I am a sister. I am a friend. I am a fighter. I am a cancer survivor."

—KIM KASS, INSPIRATION

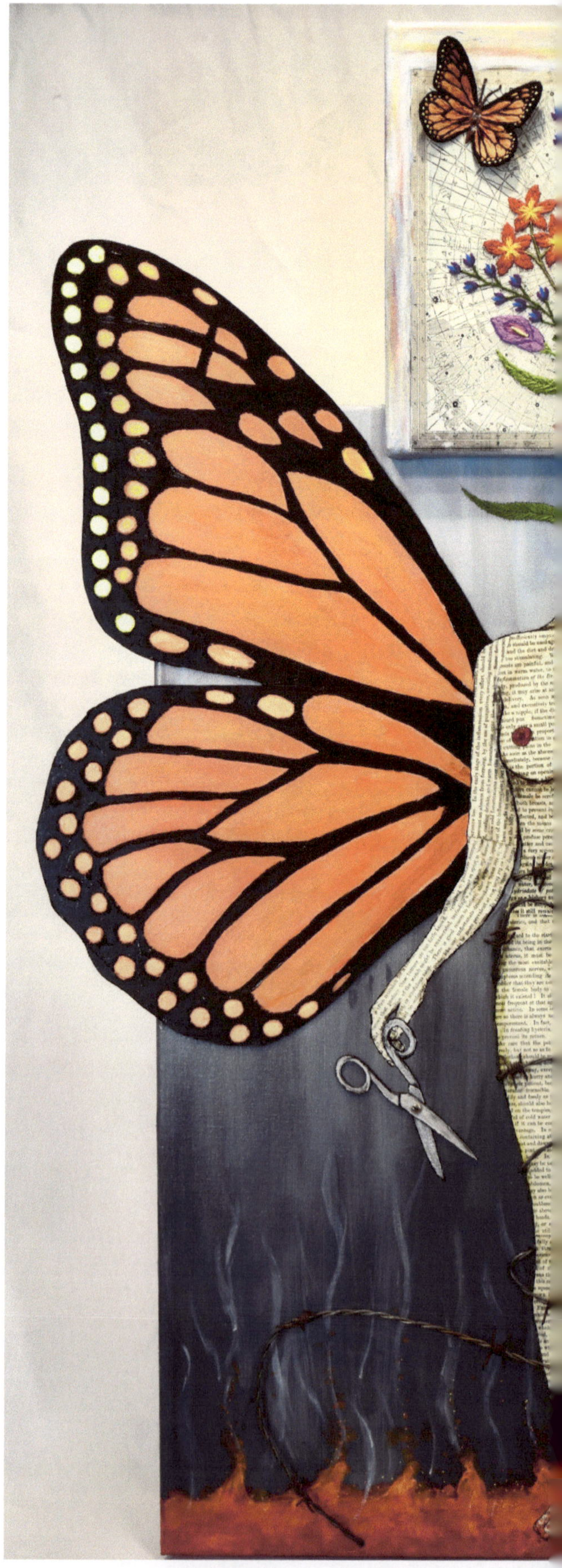

"All'alba Vincero"

Inspiration: Kim Kass
Artist: Amanda Walker

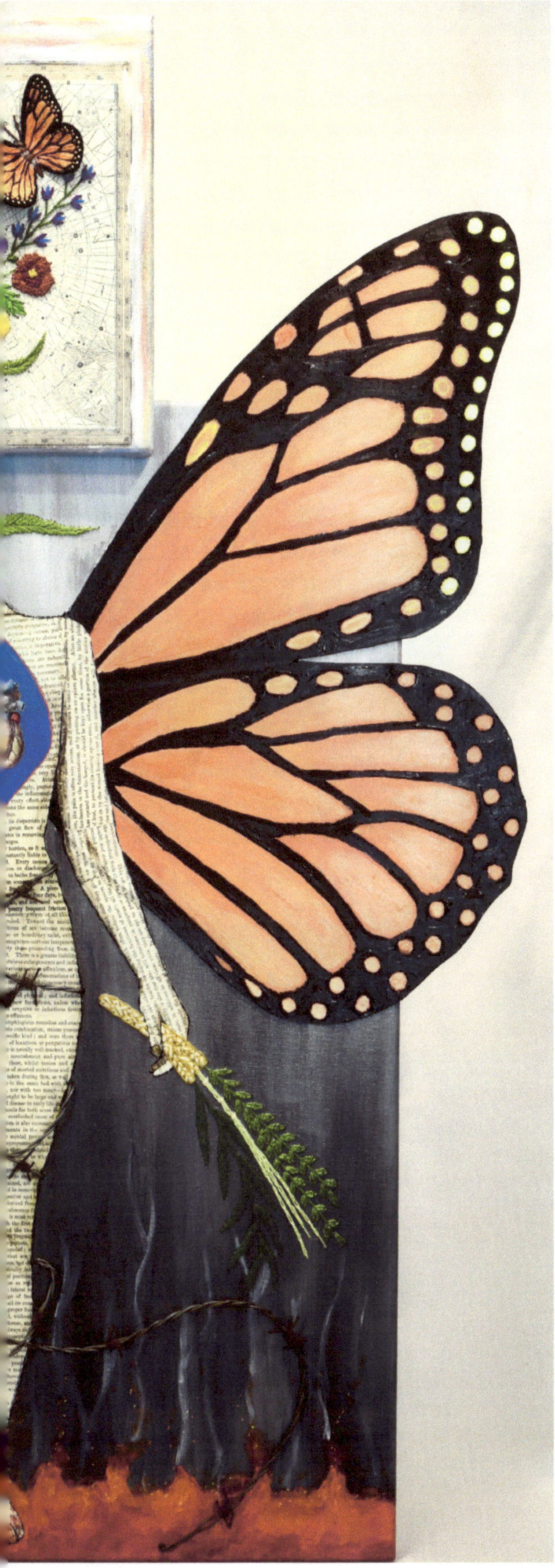

"Making this artwork to tell Kim Kass's story has been an honor for me. Kim compared having breast cancer and chemotherapy as like "being in a volcano," and that was the starting point for the piece: a figure rising out of a volcanic and smoky hell. Every image here was inspired by her story of fear, love, faith, determination, and bravery.

The text in this piece is from an original 1878 medical textbook, the star map is an original from 1903, and the eyes are Kim's. The embroidery was done by hand.

Kim told me that the central message of her piece should be "cancer will not defeat me;" and there is no doubt that such a strong figure with such powerful wings, so much determination, and so much love, will pull free of the volcano."

—AMANDA WALKER, ARTIST

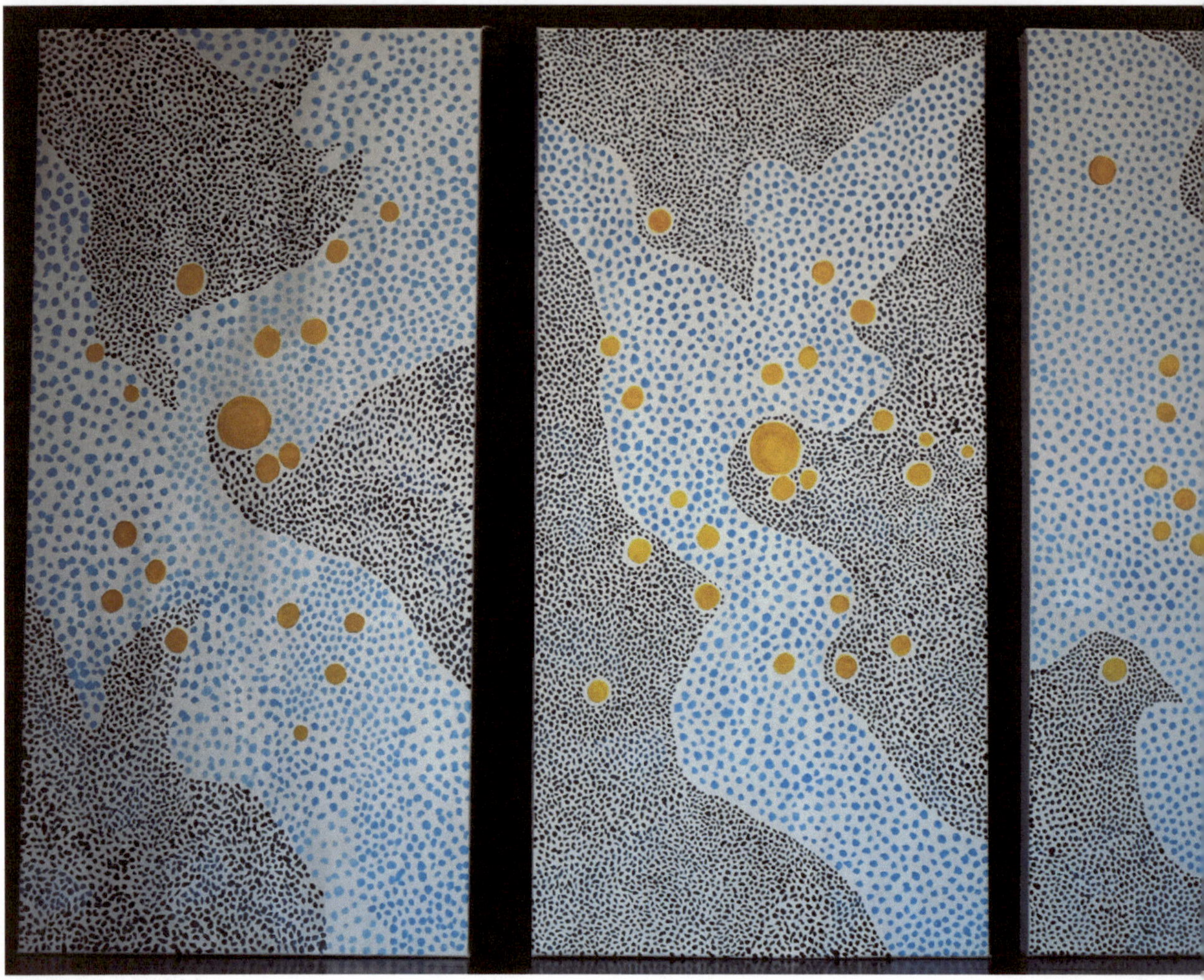

"Where the Light Enters You" **BWC Philadelphia, 2019**

Inspiration: Devon Messner (In Loving Memory)
Artist: Marie McGrory

"I truly believe everything in life happens for a reason. Lung cancer chose me. A cancer diagnosis has a way of transforming your entire being. I'm not the same person today that I was before my cancer diagnosis. I allowed cancer to change me. What was meant to destroy me- actually made me an even better version of myself. On March 1st 2018, the phone call came that changed the course of my life forever. I was at work at the time and, after the initial shock faded, I allowed myself a short cry. I realized that there was only one thing to do: WIN! Having a positive attitude is a major factor in getting yourself through a cancer diagnosis. My journey took me through brain surgery, a round of chemotherapy, and thoracic surgery to remove the primary tumor from my lung; all very necessary steps to return to a cancer-free life. From my very first meeting with my medical team, I let everyone know I was determined to beat stage 4 lung cancer. Nothing would stop me from reaching this goal. My children, Marina (15) and Michael (11), were and still are my daily inspirations. Even in the midst of a devastating disease, they were strong, supportive, and helpful. They surrounded me with their love and attention throughout the entire process. Getting to know Marie, my artist, was an extra blessing in my journey. Speaking to her about my cancer was such a freeing experience. She is one of the kindest souls I have ever met and I'm so happy to call her a friend."

—DEVON MESSNER, INSPIRATION

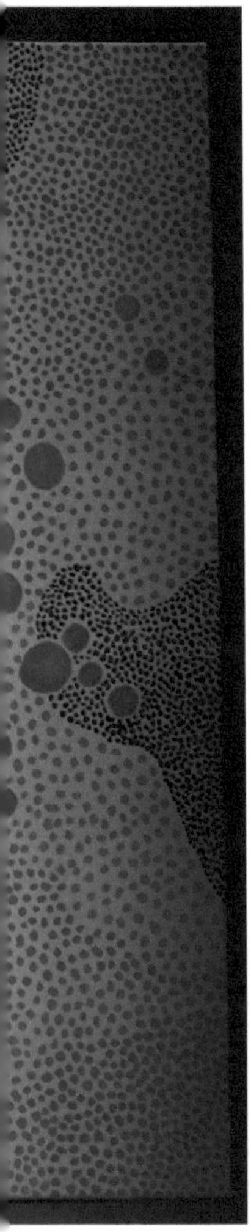

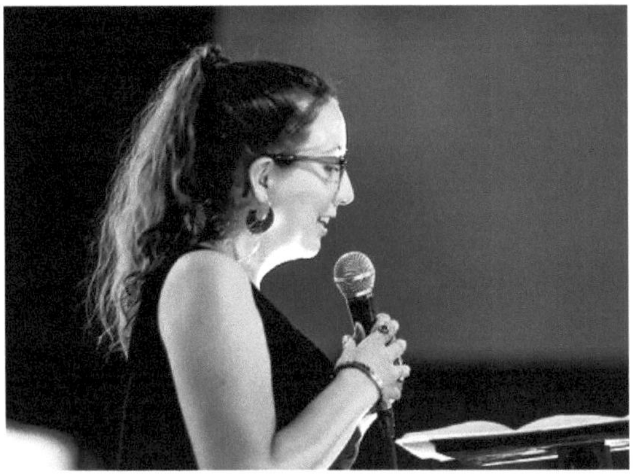

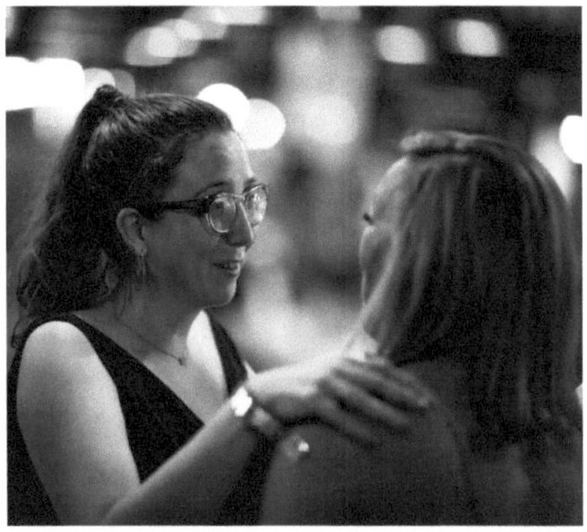

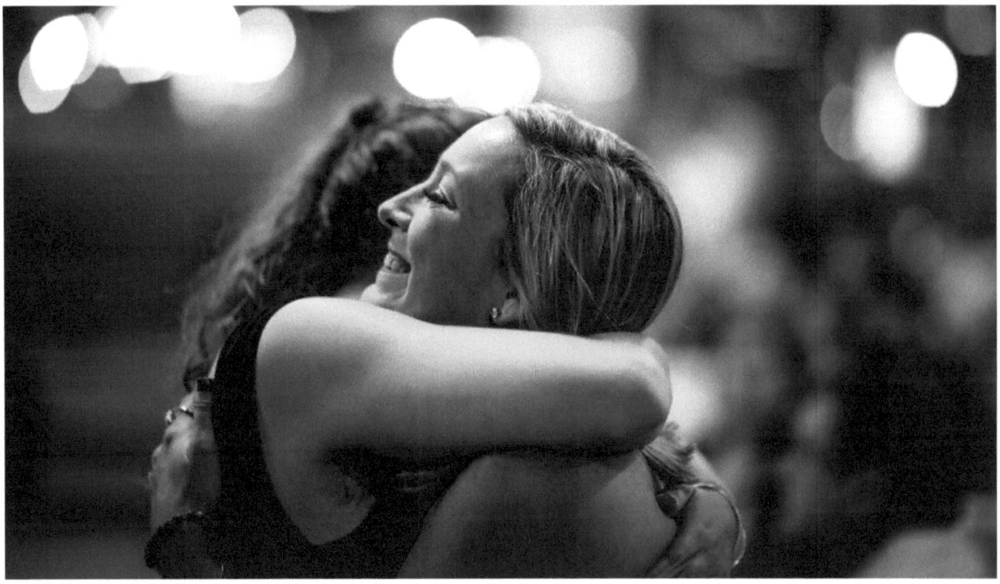

PHOTO CREDIT: ALISON CONKLIN

"Devon is a light and joy. Faced with unthinkable odds as a young mother, she fearlessly entered a time that for many, might be the darkest period of their lives, and came out stronger and brighter than ever before. During our first conversation she quoted her favorite poet, Rumi: 'The wound is the place where the light enters you.' Devon has endless light entering her, and through this experience she has changed her life for the better. Though she completed her treatment and has had clear scans for over a year, she still faced a terrifying medical anomaly this summer, requiring emergency brain surgery. Speaking to her in the days afterward, she only had good news and joy to share. She was grateful and happy and feeling good. Devon reminds me constantly that life is full of light and dark times, represented by the blues in this triptych. We may never know when the next dark wave is coming. But Devon and her light glows and grows as it pulls the good people in her life closer to her orbit. The yellow circles in this painting represent Devon and her constellation of loved ones. Through the dark waves they grow bigger and closer than ever. Today we celebrate in the light times ahead."

—MARIE MCGRORY, ARTIST

"I was 29 years old when I found out that I had cancer, and it was quite the shock to not just me, but my family and friends as well. When you receive a cancer diagnosis, you learn two things: you're stronger than you could have ever imagined and loved more than you know. Sure, there were some days when I felt I just couldn't go on and depression got the best of me. But when I look back I realize cancer wasn't a death sentence, it was a life sentence; it pushed me to live. It was one of the biggest life events I had ever experienced and I now realize how important it is to treat both your mental and physical health. I kept focusing on the 'todays' and kept remembering why I was fighting; it was so I could have more 'tomorrows.' I was not about to let an invisible enemy like cancer take me down. That determination took me to the next day and the day after that until I made it today. I kept my sense of humor with me the whole time; laughter and sarcasm was truly my best medicine. I keep sharing my story so that eventually it can help someone else get through their struggle. I've learned to have pride in how far I have come, and to have faith in how far I can go."

—COLLEEN CONNELLY, INSPIRATION

"Falling into the enormity of Colleen's smile, I found a multi layered universe of love. This image was born within my heart's eye, as I listened to the stories of her husband Pete's constant love, and the love from her parents, her extended family, her friends, her medical teams, her sports teams, her colleagues and her faith. Layers upon layers. Some seen, some unseen."

—MICHELE KELLNER, ARTIST

"Colleen's Grace"

Inspiration: Colleen Connelly
Artist: Michele Kellner

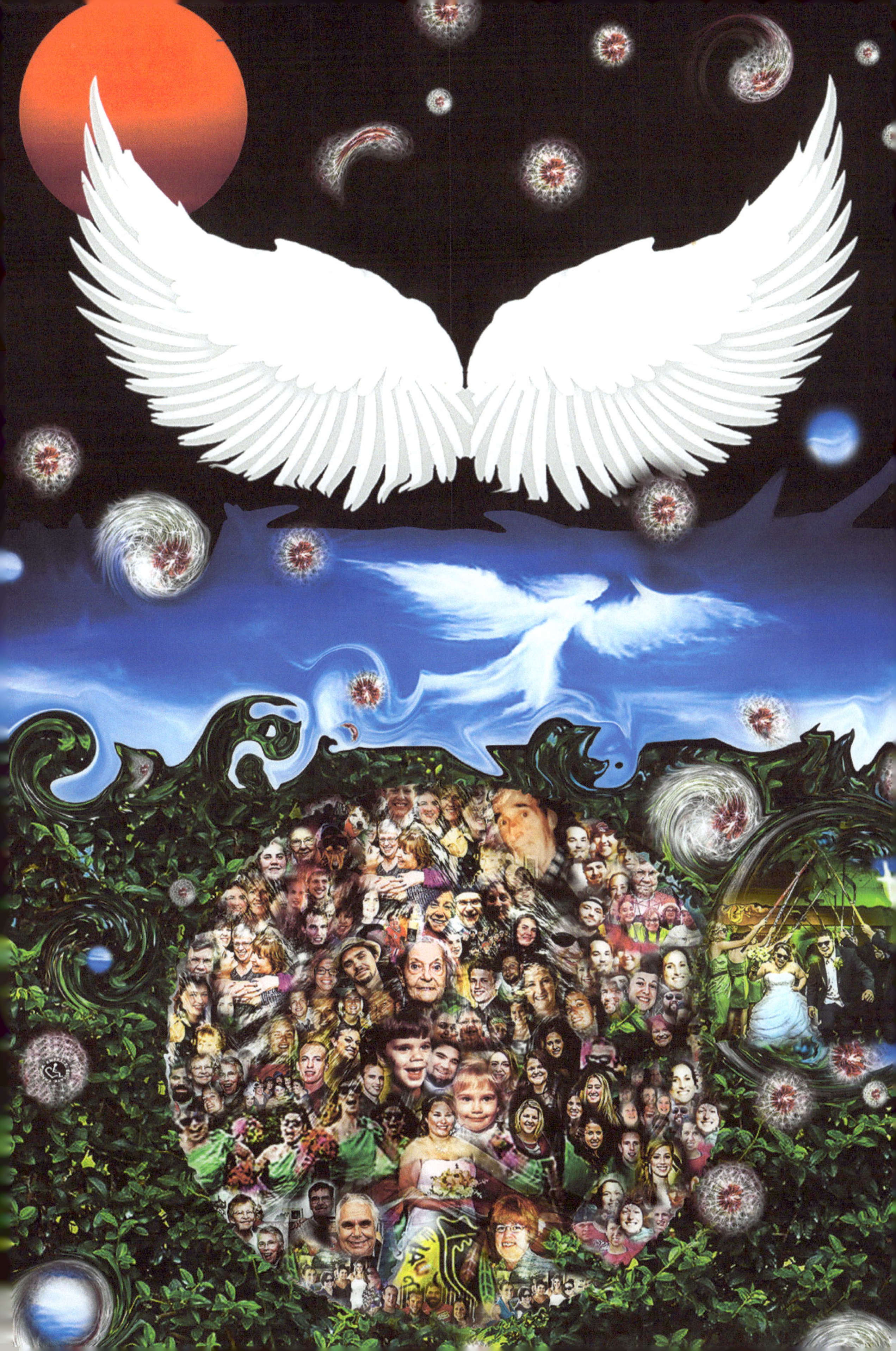

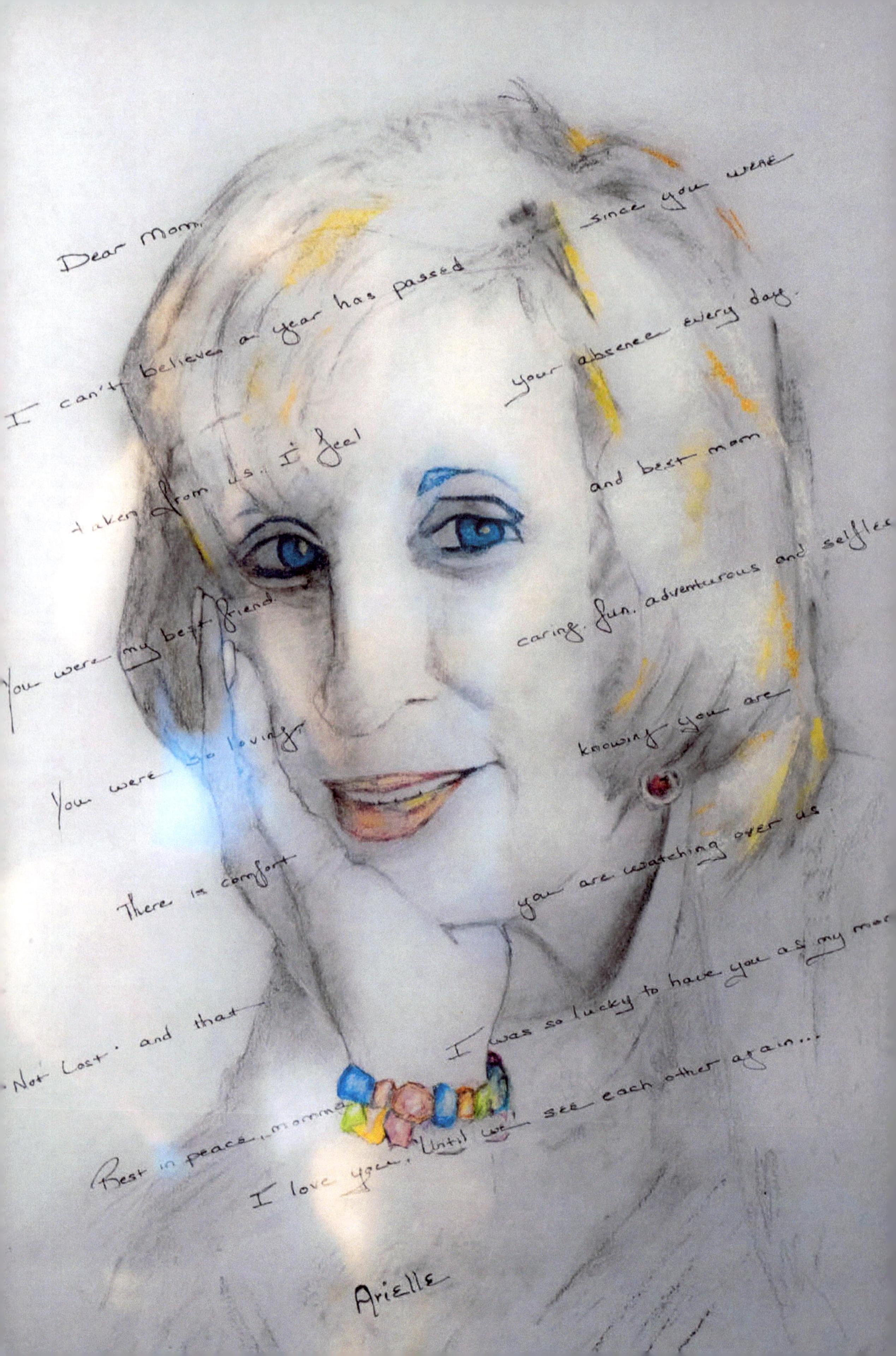
Dear Mom,
I can't believe a year has passed since you were
taken from us. I feel your absence every day.
You were my best friend and best mom
You were so loving, caring, fun, adventurous and selfless
There is comfort knowing you are
Not Lost. and that you are watching over us.
I was so lucky to have you as my mom
Rest in peace, momma
I love you. Until we see each other again...
Arielle

"My mother was diagnosed with pancreatic cancer in May 2020 and in less than four weeks, she passed. Due to COVID, we haven't been able to have a proper ceremony for her and I have been carrying such guilt about it - she deserves better. I was partnered with Ruth, and for her piece she wanted me to write a letter that made me focus on my feelings. As I wrote, I felt a weight was lifted and was able to get some closure."

—ARIELLE PRICHARD, CAREGIVER TO MOTHER

"It has been a privilege to be an artist for Brushes With Cancer. It became clear as I began working with my partner Arielle that the piece we would create would be an homage to her mom, who had recently died of pancreatic cancer, and that it would be part of her mom's memorial service. As Arielle told me about her relationship with her mom she made her mom come alive. I felt her mom's sparkle and energy and the deep and loving relationship between them. I suggested Arielle write a love letter to her mom and that we incorporate her words into the piece of art. And so we did. After I selected the photo I wanted to use for the piece, I learned that it was taken at the same venue that was selected for her mom's memorial service. Arielle and I also discovered that her mom's Hebrew name and my name were the same. Clearly, this collaboration was meant to be."

—DR. RUTH MAYER, ARTIST

"Mom"

Inspiration: Arielle Prichard
Artist: Dr. Ruth Mayer

BWC Chicago, 2021

Capturing Jenna

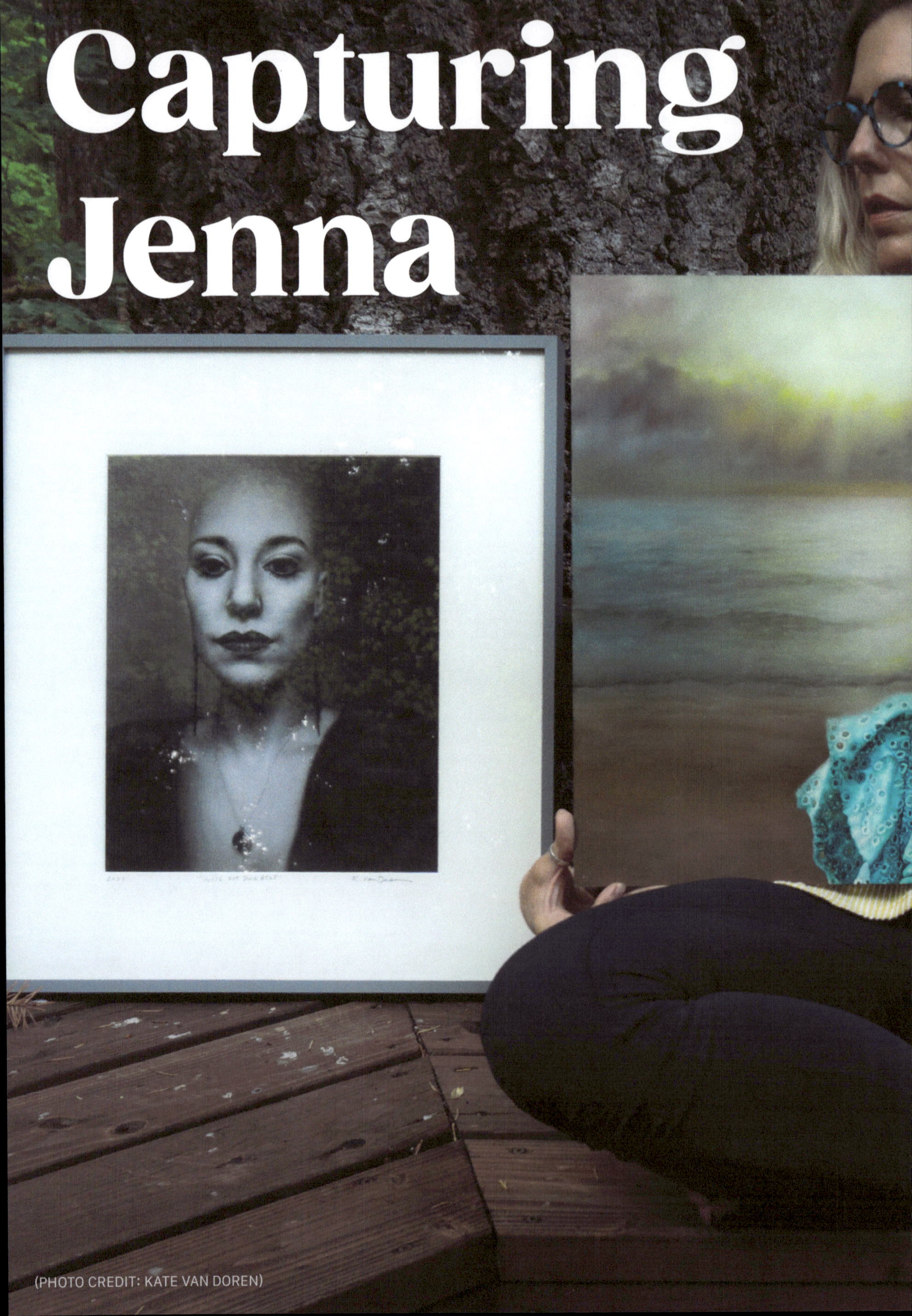

(PHOTO CREDIT: KATE VAN DOREN)

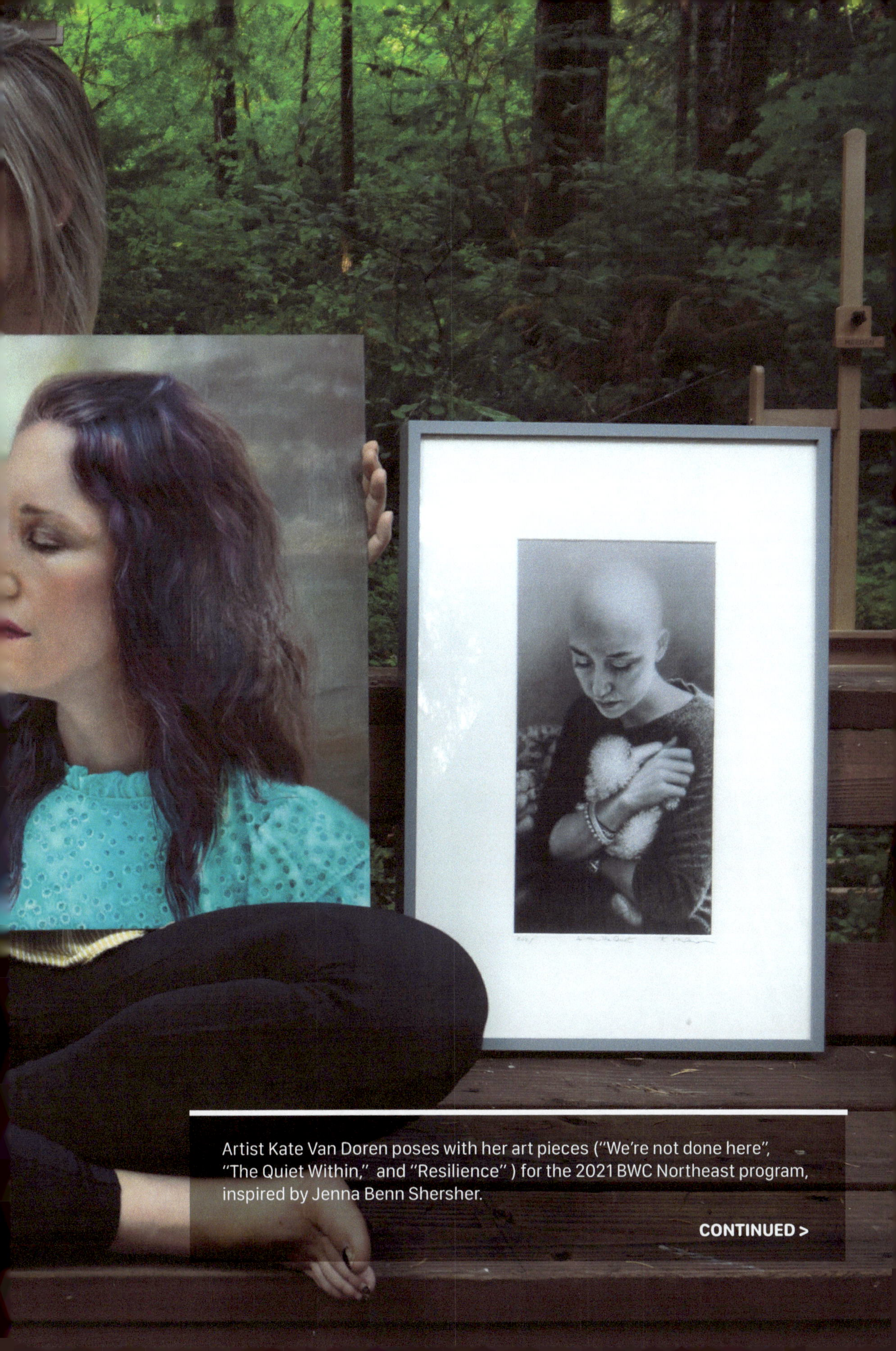

Artist Kate Van Doren poses with her art pieces ("We're not done here", "The Quiet Within," and "Resilience") for the 2021 BWC Northeast program, inspired by Jenna Benn Shersher.

CONTINUED >

The Beginning, Middle, and Now

Twist Out Cancer Founder and CEO Jenna Benn Shersher had no intention in participating as an Inspiration for Brushes with Cancer's 10th anniversary. But Artist Kate Van Doren convinced her otherwise.

"I was immediately inspired by Jenna and when I reached out to her initially about her being an Inspiration, she said no," Kate said. "She said 'I don't want to take away from someone else.'"

Kate, however, knew how significant this milestone is for Twist Out Cancer and its founder and reminded her of the courage it took to build an organization while staring cancer right in the face. The fact that Jenna is here, cancer-free, with two beautiful daughters and an organization that has touched over 140,000 globally is momentous.

"Everything Jenna touches is magic, with her empathy and ability to connect," Van Doren said. "My goal with my art is to touch others, and that's what Brushes with Cancer does."

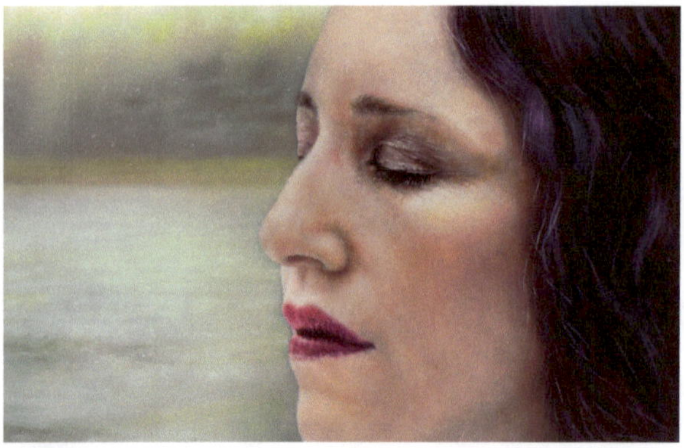

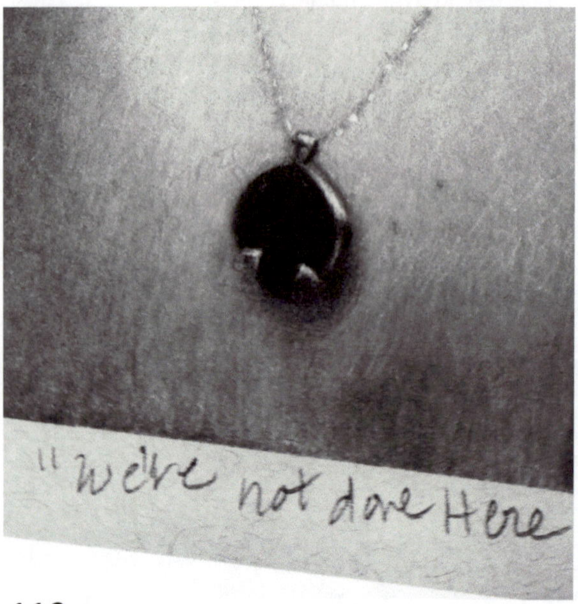

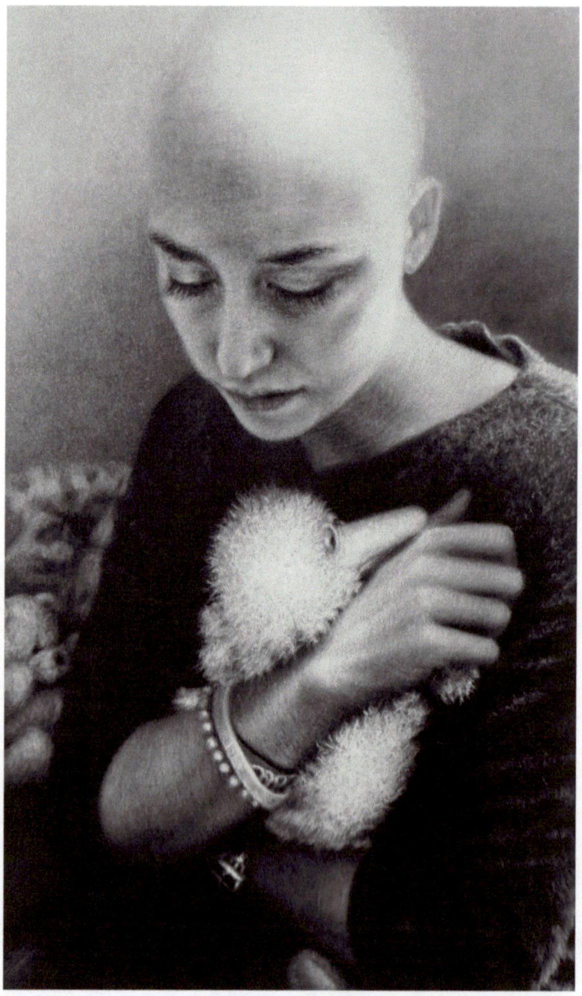

PHOTO CREDIT: KATE VAN DOREN

After Jenna agreed to be a 2021 Brushes with Cancer Inspiration, with Kate as her Artist, the two got down to business. As a 2020 Brushes with Cancer participant, Kate was already familiar with Jenna's story. There was, however, so much more for Kate to explore.

As she was doing her research, Kate discovered a few reference images that struck her. The first is one of a bald Jenna holding tight to a stuffed animal. It was the moment she learned she was cancer free. This image inspired the charcoal drawing "Within the Quiet."

"It really spoke to me," she said. "When you have cancer as a woman, you don't know if you are going to have children. So much is stripped away and you have to cling onto hope. I chose to draw this because it spoke to me in terms of the struggle women go through that isn't talked about much. When I saw that photo, I cried and was thinking about Jenna and what an incredible mother she is."

This past March, Jenna gave birth to her second daughter, Lou. A feat with its own challenges.

"I watched Jenna get the COVID vaccine while pregnant, have a baby during the pandemic and go on maternity leave while still doing her magic. It felt powerful to me to capture that."

That strength is what inspired Kate's second piece, a charcoal drawing titled "We're Not Done Here." The reference image was taken the same day Jenna learned her cancer-free news. In stark contrast, Jenna is dressed up, looking straight ahead with determination.

"My goal with my art is to touch others, and that's what Brushes with Cancer does."

—KATE VAN DOREN, ARTIST

"Jenna is one the most stunning women – she has this grace about her, but she has this fierceness and perseverance."

For the third piece – an oil painting of Jenna – Kate got in touch with Michele, the mother of one of Jenna's best friends to gather more information.

Kate was struck by an image Michelle took shortly after Jenna finished her cancer treatment. Jenna's two best friends took care of her while she was sick and once Jenna started to regain strength, they all went to the beach. The day – and the photo – are incredibly significant to Jenna, so Kate used the scene as a background in "Resilience."

In front of the beach is a side profile of a content-looking Jenna with her eyes closed, taking in how far she has come in her journey.

After spending years tackling some of life's toughest obstacles, Jenna chose to move forward with peace and healing. And instead of keeping it to herself, she has opened herself up to the world and made a tremendous impact.

"It is an incredible honor to be a part of this and what she's created," Van Doren said. "I've never seen a program like it – it's the epitome of art therapy."

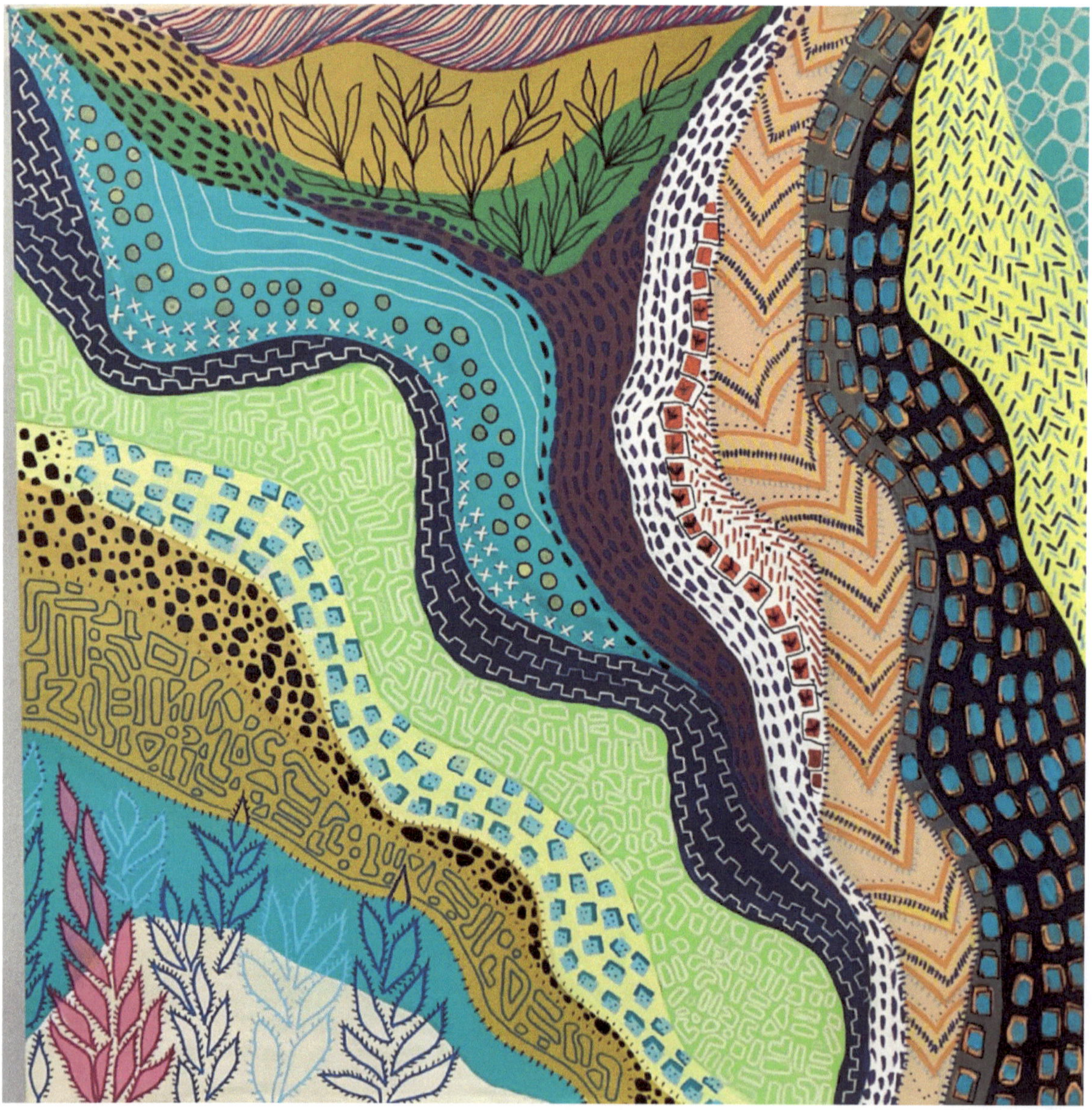

"Paper Cranes For Pam"

Inspiration: Pam Crowther
Artist: Jacqueline Carmody

BWC Southern, 2022

Finding the Good in Life's Challenges

As many of us do, Pam Crowther remembers words of wisdom from her parents. Her mom once said, "Find the good in life's challenges and always be thankful for what God has provided." Pam recalled this in 2003 when she heard those life changing words, "You have cancer."

Her chemotherapy treatments for breast cancer became "happy hours" with her friends. She hosted a wig and head shaving party and ran and participated in several marathons. She found a way to make a difficult experience a positive one and used every bit of her time to laugh and cherish life and friendship. She has since used her experience as a survivor to redirect her energy to a place of hope. Following her mom's advice, Pam only found a way to heal herself but also give back to a community that has become an extension of her own family.

Then Pam found out about Twist Out Cancer's Brushes with Cancer program from her friend, Kim Kass, a Twist Out Cancer Board Member who was also an Inspiration.

For the 2022 Southern Brushes With Cancer program, Pam was paired with Jacqueline Carmody, an accomplished artist, Board Member, and employee at Twist. They instantly connected and Jackie was blown away with how Pam owns her story for life so proudly.

"The artwork that I created for Pam is called 'Paper Cranes' because she had been given origami paper cranes during her treatment by a supporting staff on her team," Jacqueline said. The paper cranes serve as a symbol for the support network in Pam's life, but also for her flexibility throughout her treatment. Pam chose to make the best of each moment throughout her treatment, and truly turned something flat into a beautiful, unique, and interesting experience. Much like one does when creating an origami figure from a flat piece of paper."

Going through the Brushes with Cancer experience, Pam learned that healing can come from being vulnerable, while opening up and sharing her story. She also saw how the connection with Jacqueline led to a friendship where they both listened to each other's stories.

Upon reflecting on her Brushes with Cancer experience, Pam said, "It's touching, it's humbling, and very emotional for me to know that someone else cares about my story. I appreciate that Jackie was drawn to my story and is creating this art piece that I will be able to see and know that is my lifelong story. It brings me to tears."

"I feel like there can be so many 'twists' to cancer, even in one person's story. My cancer journey - from diagnosis to surgery, chemotherapy, radiation and surgery again and all the emotions that came with all that - was made tolerable and at times so beautiful with the love and support of my God, my family, my friends, my church, my therapy horse, my children as my medicine and my husband firmly planted by my side. I learned that I had to fight to be my own advocate. I had to do my own research and learned that despite their best intentions, some doctors have their own agenda, which could put my health and wellbeing at risk. I learned that my voice had to rise above and be louder and stronger than all the rest of the noise. And there was a lot of noise!

But, another twist is that cancer would not be my last battle. It would not even be my most difficult one. Shortly after treatment ended, one month to be exact, my family entered another battle ring. I know beyond a shadow of a doubt that I made it through cancer treatment so that I could be here for this one. There was a purpose and a plan all along for the strengthened bonds with my family during that cancer journey—proof of a loving God who goes before and paves a way."

—JENNIFER KING, INSPIRATION

"The image is of a superhero mounted on her steed, charging in to save the day. If you look closely, you can see within the horse's determined eye is a church, which will forever be the direction these heroes will look for their salvation. As an artist, I use imagery to portray emotion and tell a story. I create large-scale, multi-media art you can feel - not just emotionally, but also physically. This piece uses a trompe l'oeil to create depth, and incorporates tactile elements of physical fur you can pet and reigns you can touch.

When I met Jennifer, I found her to be un-humanly kind, graceful, strong, and eloquent. Her experience with cancer was extremely isolating. While getting to know her story I asked, 'What was the biggest take-away from your experience?' She replied that 'my children gave me purpose.'

I've illustrated her as a valiant archer resembling the Greek goddess Artemis, goddess of the hunt and protector of children, and adorned in her children's favorite colors. The horse she rides is a stylized version of her real therapy horse named Archer.

The title of this artwork is 'Artemis.' I believe Jennifer King is a current day goddess and we should all strive to be more like her in our everyday lives. In true Jennifer King style, she's taken her experience and decided to become an advocate for others! Her aim is to educate people of ALL the recovery options available after surviving a fight with breast cancer."

—ERIN GREGANTI, ARTIST

"Artemis"

Inspiration: Jennifer King
Artist: Erin Greganti

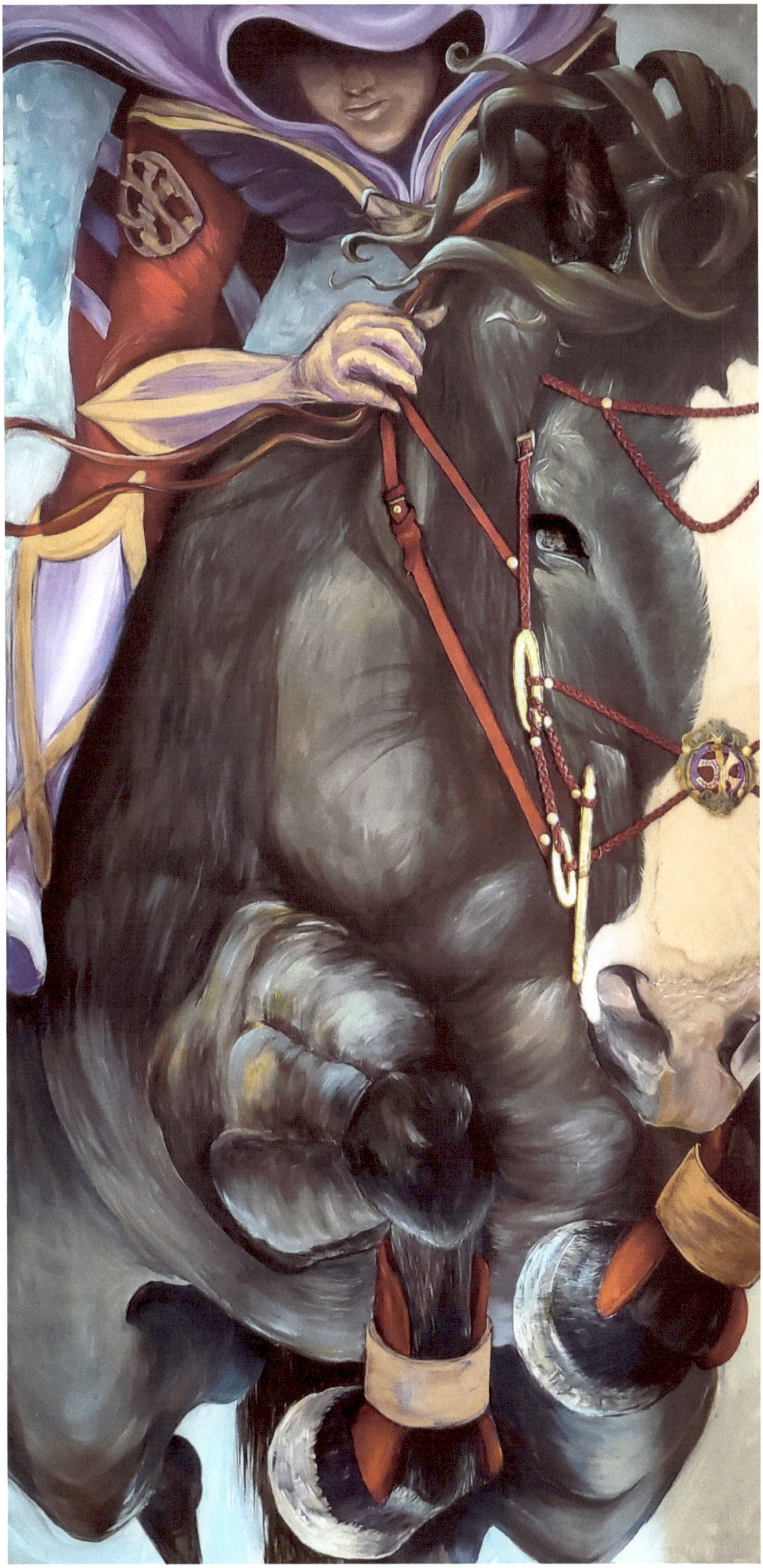

"Cancer for me was about acceptance and a willingness to do so. I learned that you have to let others mourn the way they want to and in that you gift them what they need. My eyes were opened to a first hand experience of the trials and tribulations of being a nurse. They deserve the most respect.

—EYAL SCHECTER, INSPIRATION

"This photo collage represents what a new dawn would feel like to my Inspiration, Eyal. While going through chemotherapy - in spite of the terrible side effects and the specific horrific sensations of itching and scratching - Eyal was thinking about the day after he would get a clean bill of health. He wrote a To Do List of goals that would enable him to start a new and fulfilling life in Florida. This day arrived! A CT scan indicated that Eyal is now cancer-free and can make his dream a reality."

—AKIVA GROSS, ARTIST

"Dawn"

Inspiration: Eyal Schecter
Artist: Akiva Gross

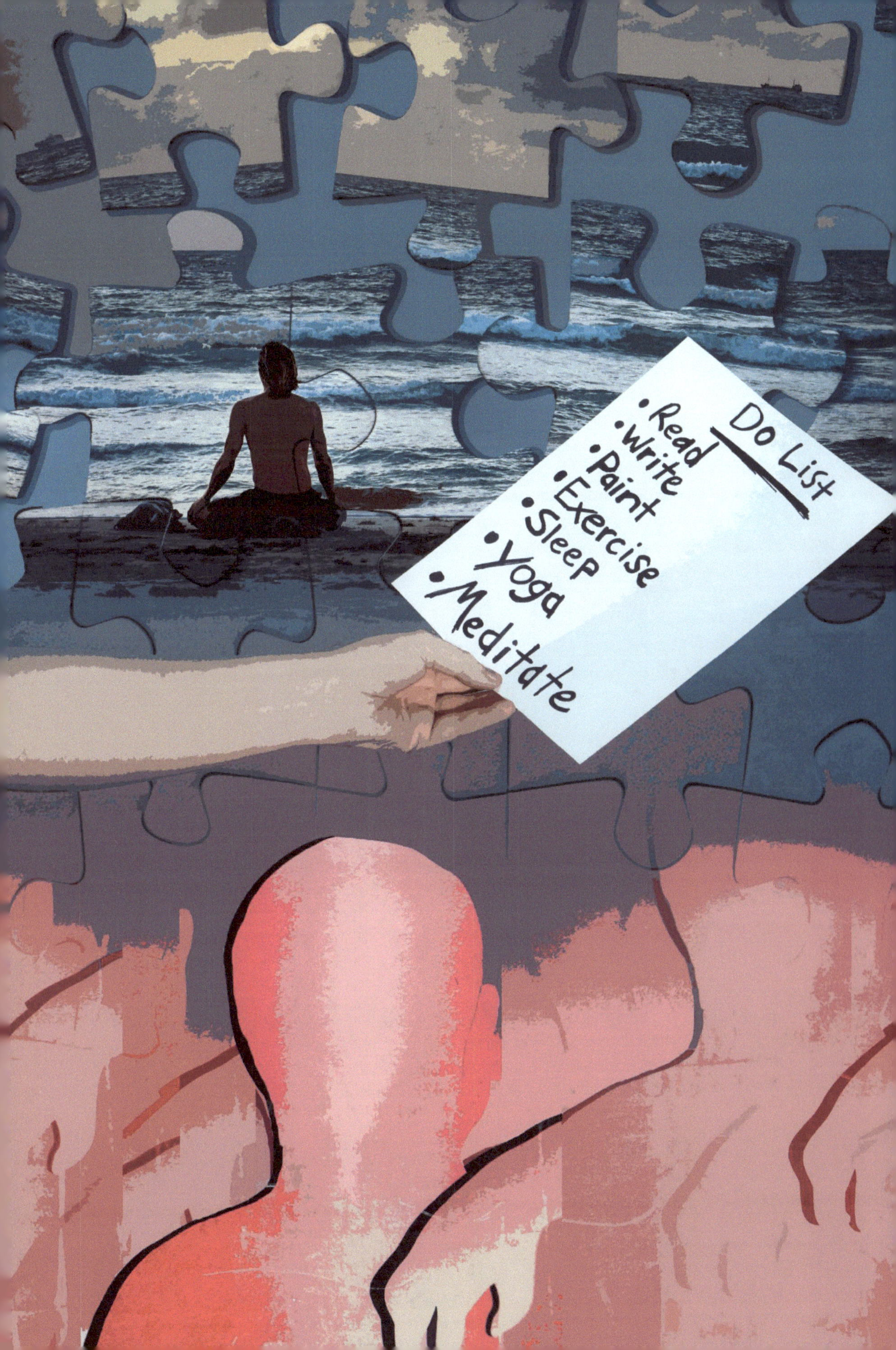
Do List
• Read
• Write
• Paint
• Exercise
• Sleep
• Yoga
• Meditate

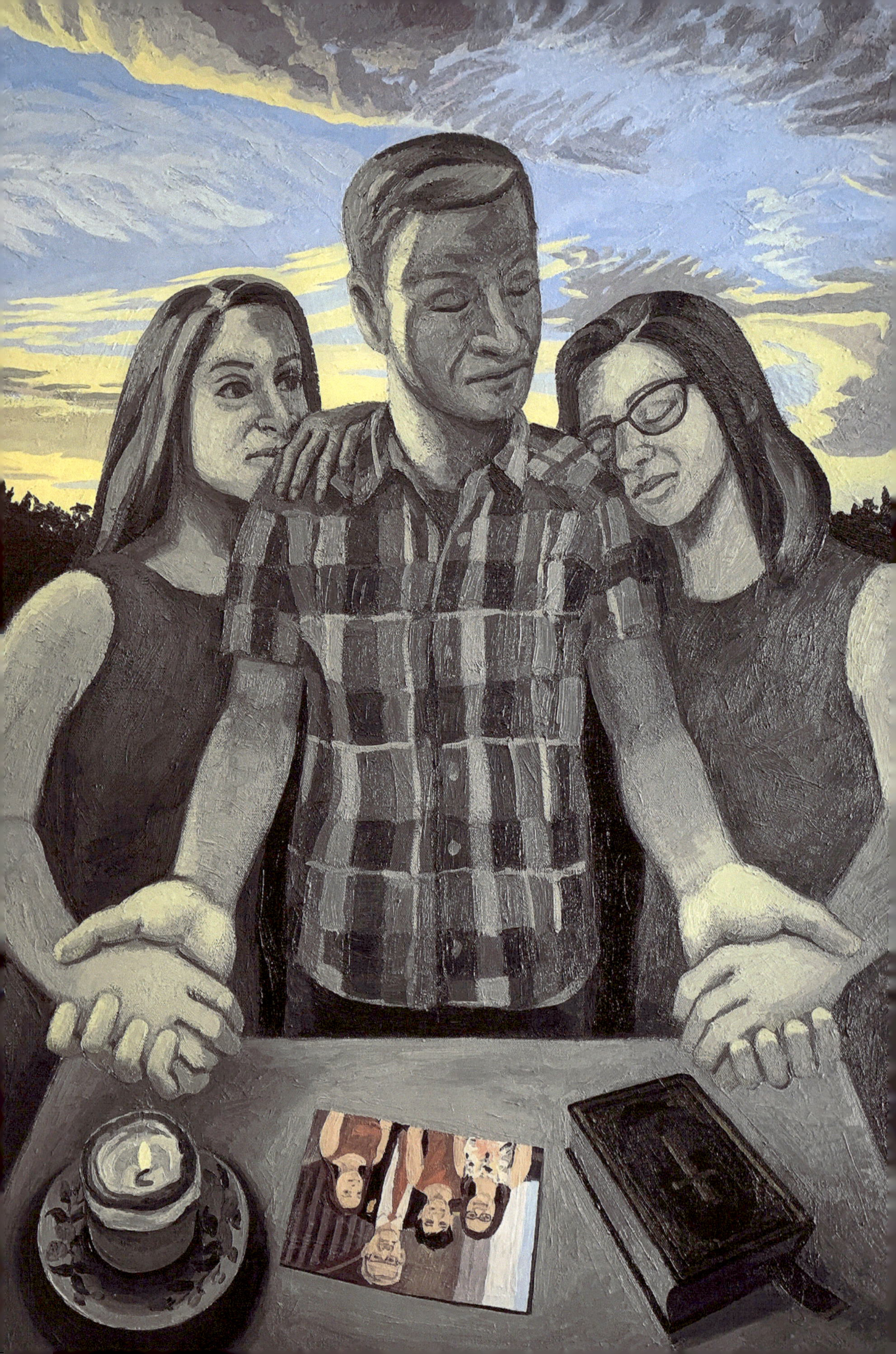

"CANCER is a dream buster!!! Cancer is the devil!!! Cancer sucks!!!

Being a caregiver is no easy ride. I questioned myself many times. There's so much information about cancer that's thrown in your lap. From one caregiver to another, my advice is to maintain a positive attitude. I know it's not always easy, especially when you're trying to accommodate every need. You are mentally and physically exhausted, but positivity remains the best medicine for the one you love.

Please remember these words from Jim Valvano 'laugh, think, and cry each day, and don't give up. Don't ever give up.'

I praise all who are fighting this horrid nasty disease, including caregivers. I have gotten to know Taurus on a much deeper level during the summer. In addition to being one of the most talented artists I know Taurus has a huge big heart, a very profound understanding of how precious life is and I am glad to be able to call him my friend.

—JEFFREY FROGGETT, INSPIRATION

"From the very first conversation, Jeff was so gracious and easy to talk to. Every time we spoke, it was clear how radiant and wonderful his wife Julie was. After we had a few encounters, I knew I wanted to make a painting that dealt with loss and strength. I imagined this scene of Jeff being strong for his daughters, as they all deal with the loss of the beautiful light that Julie brought into their lives."

—TAURUS BURNS, ARTIST

"An Enduring Faith"

Inspiration: Jeffrey Froggett
Artist: Taurus Burns

"I was diagnosed with Stage II breast cancer in October of 2019, just after working on The Brushes with Cancer event for Jenna. A year later, in August of 2020, my husband was diagnosed with Stage IV lung cancer.

After learning about my husband's diagnosis, I started a fundraiser for research projects that will benefit patients like him living with EGFR lung cancer. I used my contacts in the Philadelphia dining scene and my social media savvy to propel a two-month fundraiser that brought together the public and our hospitality colleagues. We raised over $100k for two research projects for LUNGevity & EGFR resisters, which are now fully funded for 2021."

—KRISTINA BURKE, INSPIRATION

"We both believe (and have found from experience) that the more open you are and the more you share your story, resources and experience, the more the universe finds a way to give back to you. Cancer is a daily grind, it's a constant and relentless battle that requires fortitude, empathy, awareness and hopefulness. But you make connections with people along the way that fill you with a hope or a new sense of purpose. You cannot stop finding joy or sparking joy for others. As much as cancer takes from people, it can be the impetus for realizing how fragile life is, which in turn makes you appreciate small moments which can make you feel whole."

—JIM BURKE, INSPIRATION
IN LOVING MEMORY

"Love conquers all. And that is certainly the case with my inspirations, Kristina and Jim Burke. Before meeting them in person, I learned that they both were diagnosed with cancer in the past 2 years. Such a situation would be hard for most people to handle, but not for this phenomenal couple who amaze me with their strength, spirit and above all else, love for each other, their children and life and all its moments. When we met, Kristina likened her experience with cancer to being underwater – feeling both weightless and heavy with hopeful light above and unknown darkness below. As she and Jim reminisced about time spent on the coast of Italy listening to Neil Young's Harvest Moon, I envisioned a painting of them embracing in moonlight. The resulting artwork is layered, starting with their figures underwater – hers on the move, just as she is – his still, with an open ear, listening. Tender and tough, together they will be able to handle whatever comes their way."

—MAURA MATTHEWS, ARTIST

"INSIEME"

Inspirations: Kristina Burke & Jim Burke
Artist: Maura Matthews

BWC Northeast, 2021

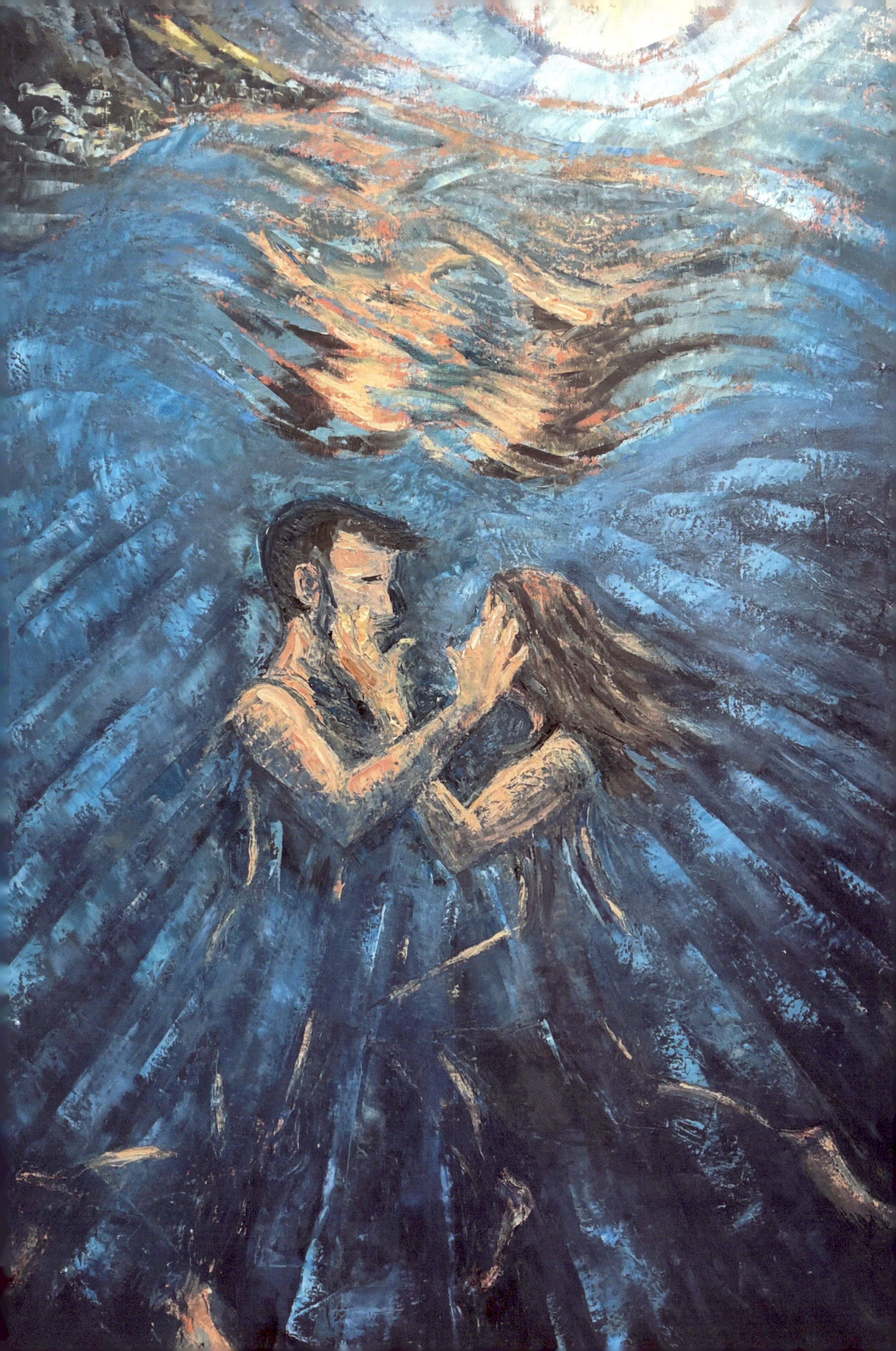

PHOTOS OF THIS SECTION PRODUCED BY THE CREATIVE VISIONS OF:

Aleya Cydney

Alison Conklin

Liesl Diesel

J&J Studios, LLC

Einav and Amit Payes

Shelby Ricci

Louis Terry

celebrate

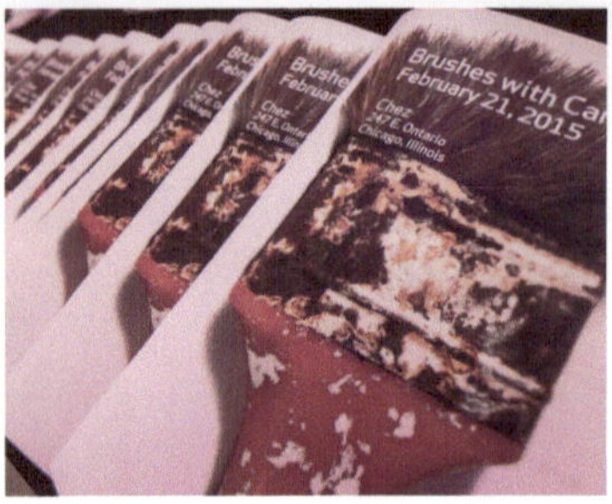

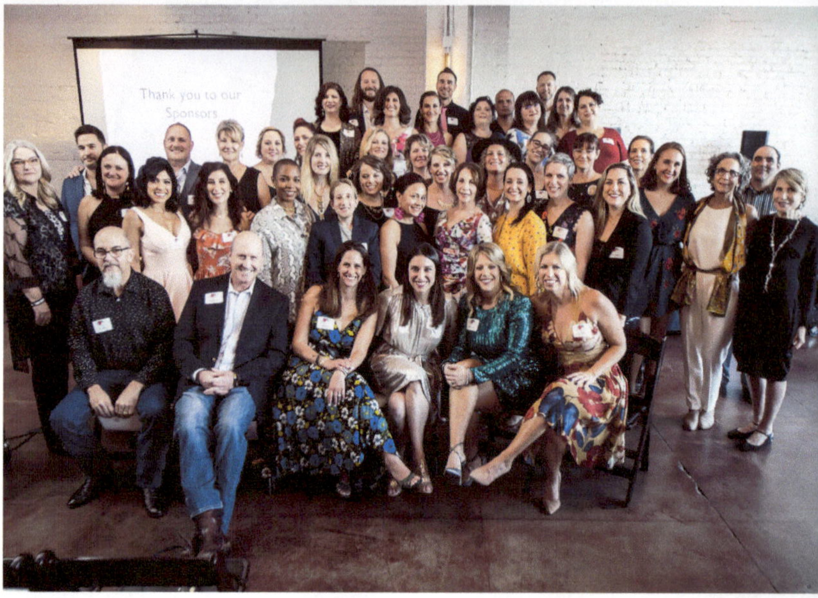

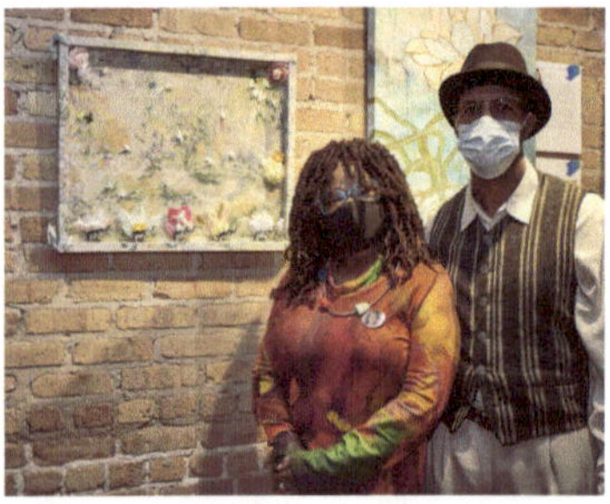

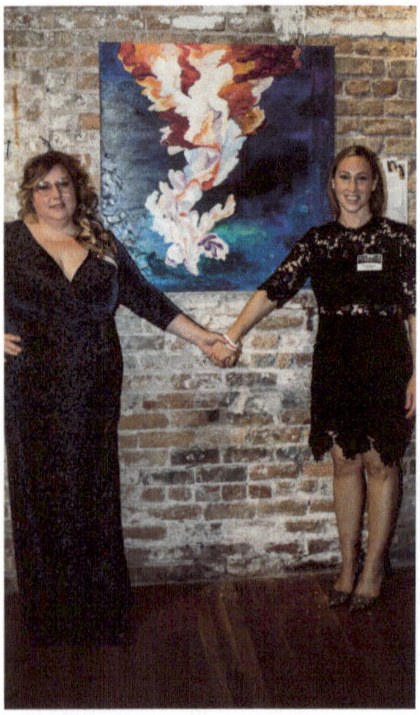

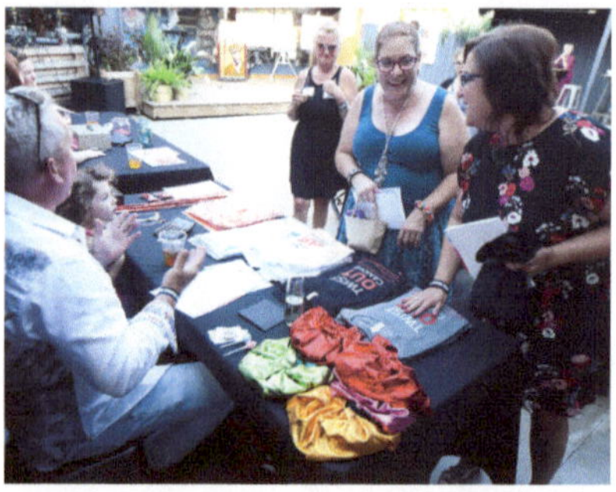

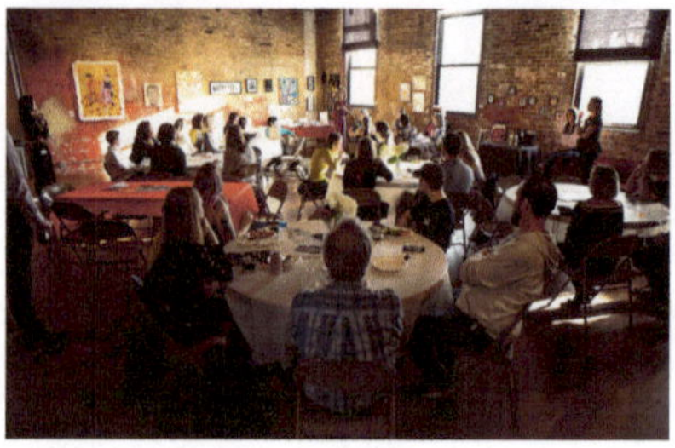

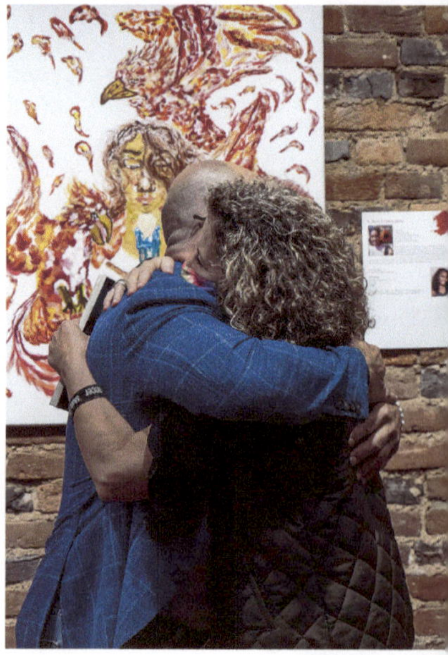

In its 10th year, Brushes with Cancer will host participants from all over the world, including the U.K., Mexico, India and Germany.

But connecting those touched by cancer internationally isn't something Jenna Benn Shersher had originally intended when she founded Twist Out Cancer 10 years ago. It was just an organic part of her life.

Prior to being diagnosed with Grey Zone Lymphoma at 29 years old, Jenna spent seven years going to school and beginning her career in Montreal. Over those years, she deeply connected with the Montreal community.

"I knew that when I finished cancer treatment, I wanted to do something there because the community

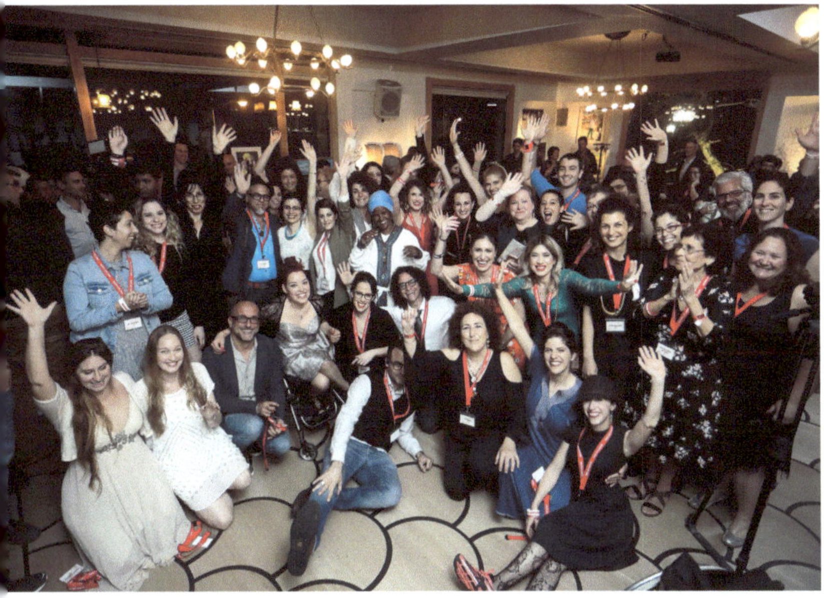

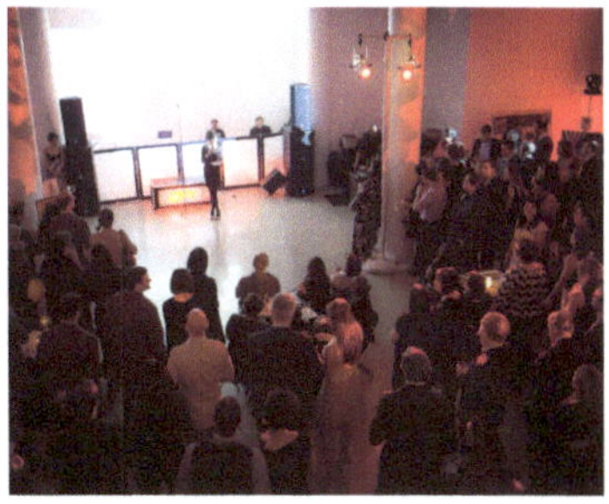

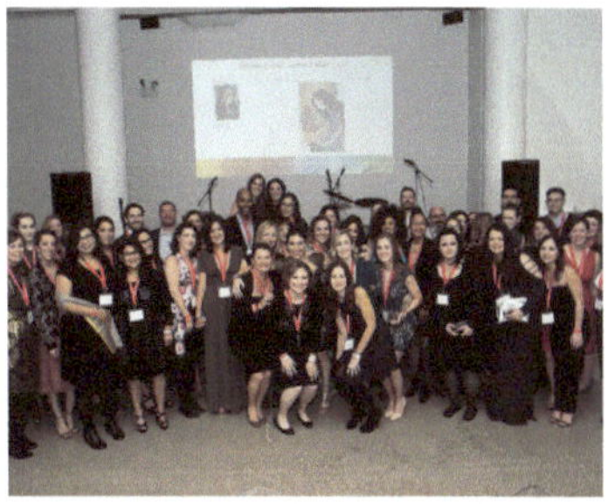

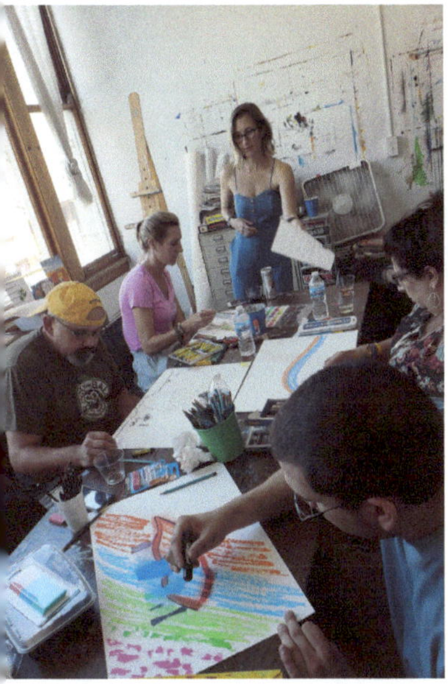

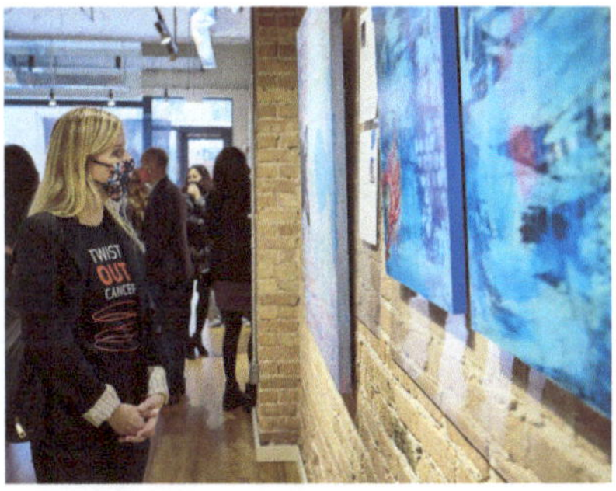

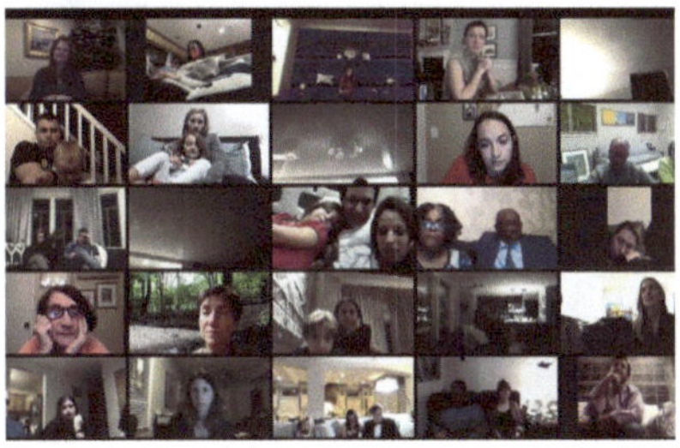

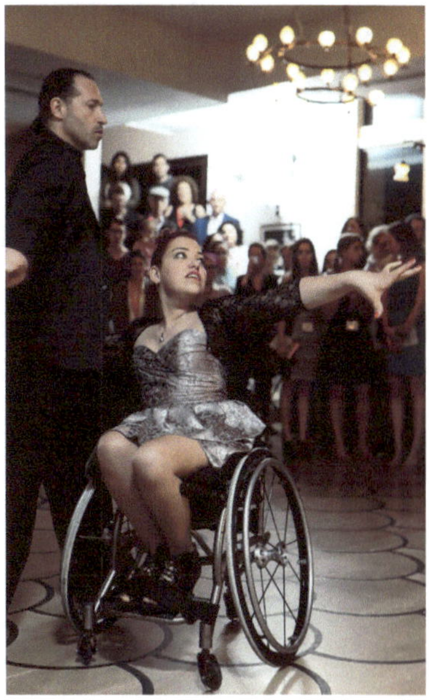

had been so supportive to me."

When Jenna became cancer free and founded Twist Out Cancer, she wanted her first fundraising event to be in Montreal. It was a night that was absolute fate. Jenna's friends learned that iconic rock musician Chubby Checker was in town for his 50th anniversary tour.

Checker's music has long been part of Jenna's life, as her father introduced her to '50s and '60s rock while she was growing up. During her cancer treatment, she did The Twist – a simple move her rapidly changing body could handle – to connect to her love of dance.

"He was this icon while I was going through treatment," she said.

Knowing how personal Checker's music is to Benn Shersher, her friends reached out to his management and pulled some strings. The night of his show, Benn Shersher was doing The Twist with the man who inspired one of the biggest moments of her life.

"It was so meaningful to me because there I was, dancing and healthy with a person who had become so significant throughout childhood, sickness and survivorship," she said. "It was a pretty out-of-body experience."

It was the perfect way to kick off Twist Out Cancer's beginning. Throughout the next 10 years, Benn Shersher, along with members of the Twist community, would connect to thousands of people touched by cancer, across a number of borders.

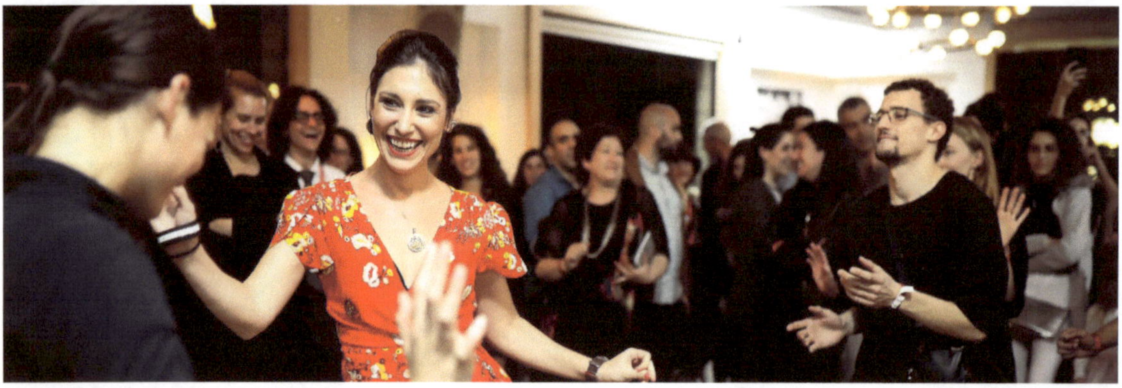

CANCER KNOWS NO BOUNDARIES

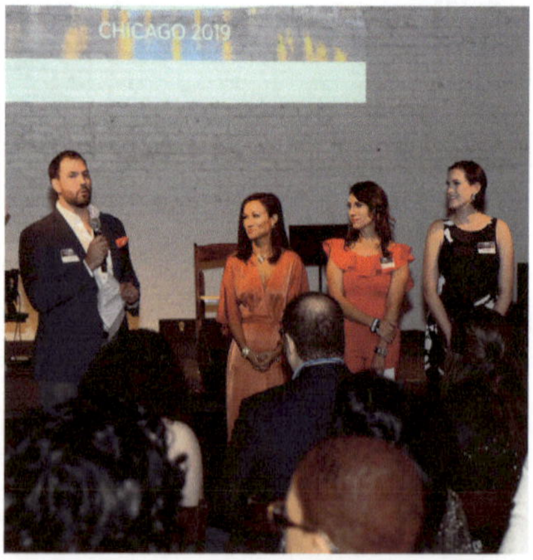

Inviting the world along to share, connect and heal seems like a big undertaking. For Jenna, it's a concept that is universal.

"Cancer knows no boundaries, so I was never intimidated about launching programs where I didn't live," she said.

The first Brushes with Cancer event took place in Chicago, a natural location for the inaugural event. Jenna grew up in the area, had family there and Chicago had been the backdrop of most of her cancer journey.

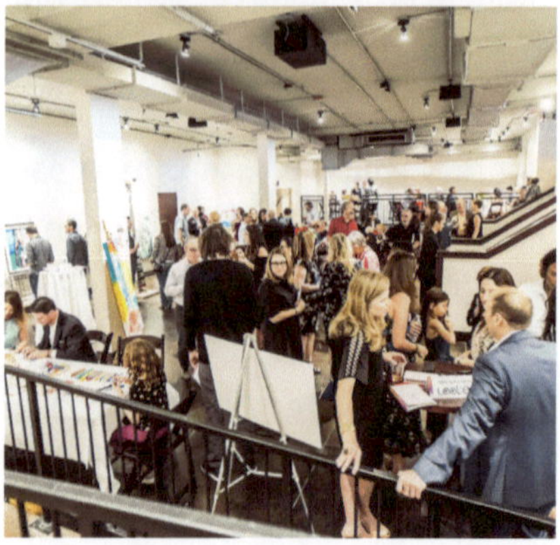

But Jenna knew she had to also honor her passion for traveling and connecting, so she began working toward hosting Brushes with Cancer programs outside of the United States. A feat that took a whole community and a lot of connecting, something Twist Out Cancer Program Director August Spree was thrilled to participate in.

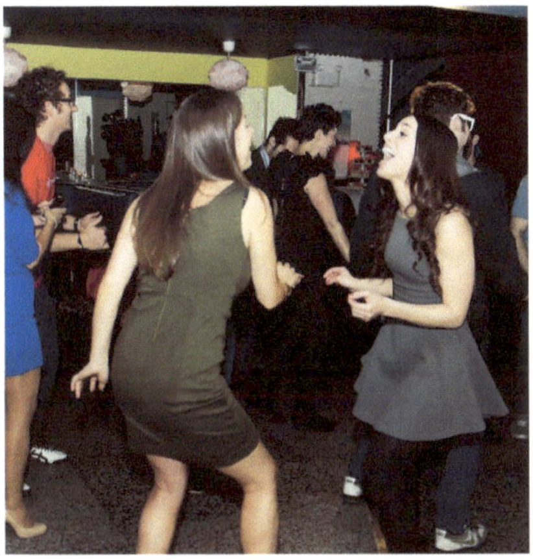

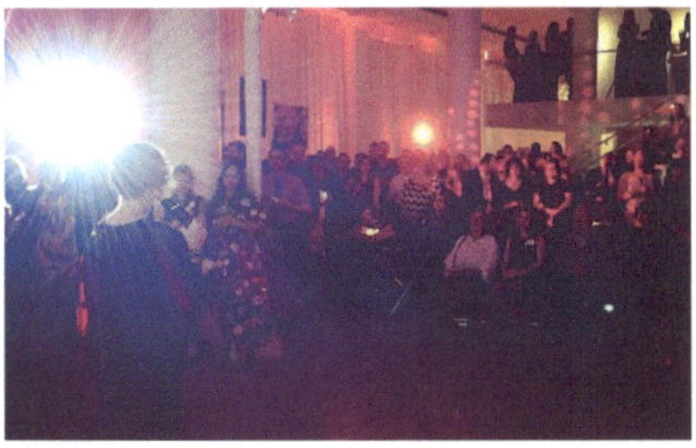

A cancer survivor, August attended a Brushes with Cancer event by chance – a chance that became life changing.

"I was like, 'This is the thing that my heart has been looking for,'" August said. "Brushes with Cancer takes points of beauty that can come from painful situations – and they're so hard to see when you're in it."

August approached Jenna and said confidently, "We are going to be friends."

It was the right place at the right time, as Jenna was in the middle of planning a Brushes with Cancer event in Israel, a special place for both women. Already, August knew of an Israeli event professional from the work she did at a youth organization that took her to the country.

Jenna found someone who could help Twist Out Cancer take the next step toward a big undertaking.

COMING FULL CIRCLE

While Israel was not Brushes with Cancer's first international experience, it was the most personal. With familial roots in Israel and her wedding taking place in Tel Aviv, it was only a matter of time before Jenna brought Brushes to a place that feels like home to her.

However, there were a healthy set of challenges to navigate.

"In Israel, the biggest impediment for me is the language," Jenna said. "Program books had to be translated into Hebrew, including video. I needed to find people on the ground that were fluent in Hebrew and English that could help with the recruitment process."

Language wasn't the only thing lost in translation. There were also cultural differences between Americans and Israelis. In Israel, it is mandatory for citizens to serve in the military once they reach 18. The experience is expected for Israelis, and also incredibly difficult.

"Parents have to essentially say goodbye to their kids and hope for the best," Jenna said.

"Sabras" – a fruit that is hard on the outside and sweet on the inside – is a colloquial term used to describe Israelis. Tough exteriors are part of the culture out of necessity.

"Giving those touched by cancer permission and a space to talk about their feelings was a unique and novel concept within Israel. To get them involved in the program required a lot of heavy lifting. We had to be strategic on how to approach it."

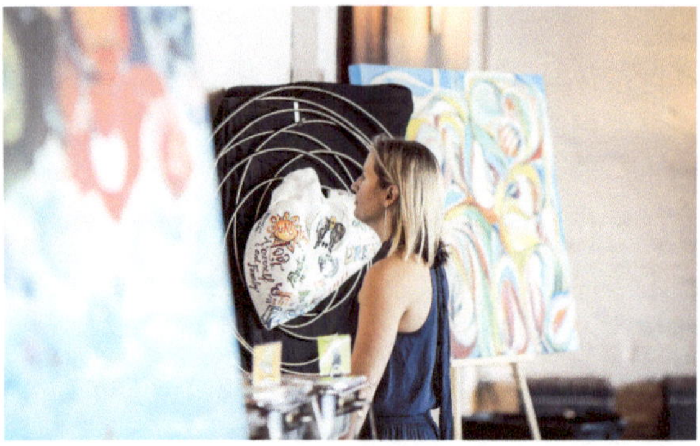

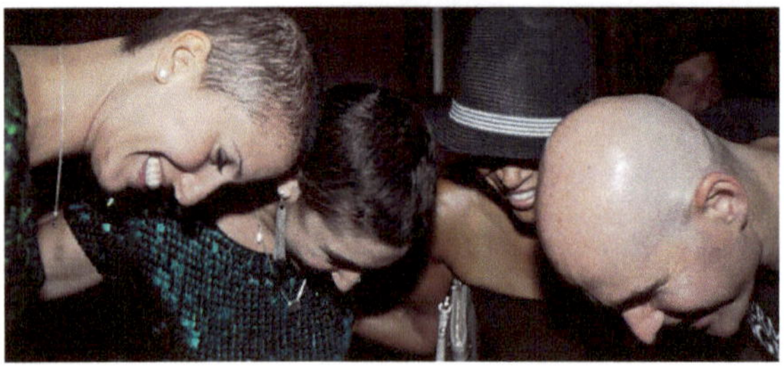

There was also the diversity in the region to navigate. Being so close to the Middle East and East African countries, the region is filled with different backgrounds, religions and ethnicities.

Jenna had support, though. During the wedding planning process, she became close with the venue owner Chen Levran, who offered up his venue the next time she needed to host an event. She did, and Jenna and her hardworking team hosted Israel's first Brushes with Cancer and in the same venue as her wedding five years prior.

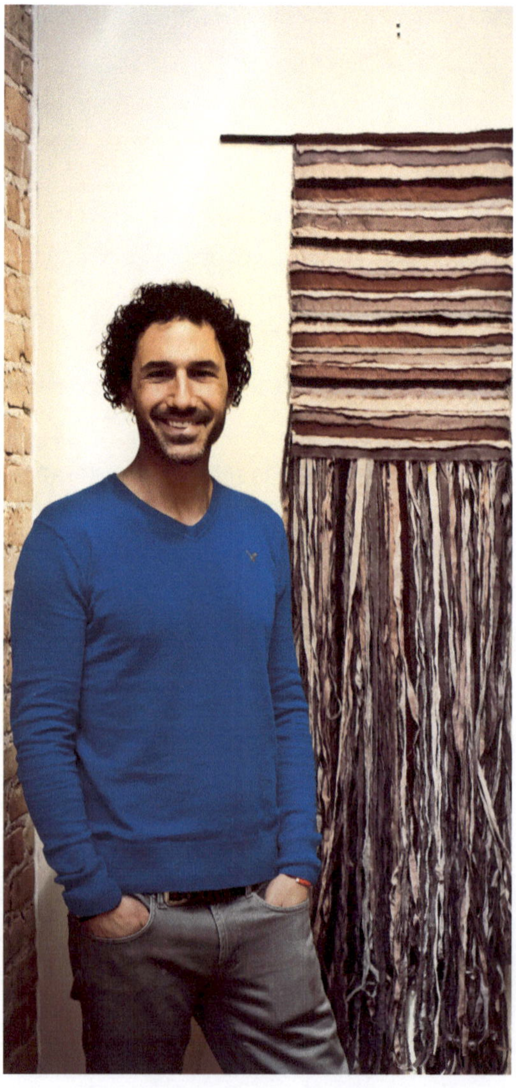

THE INTERNATIONAL GROWTH CONTINUES

As of 2022, Twist Out Cancer has held more than 23 Brushes with Cancer events in three countries. Artists and Inspirations are welcomed from all over the world, with virtual options making distance less challenging.

"Now that we're living in a virtual space, boundaries don't matter anymore," Jenna said. "Participants can be from all over the world! Up until a couple years ago, we were focused on regions and it doesn't have to stay that way."

Opening up the program internationally also invites cross-cultural conversations that never would have happened without Twist's international influence.

"So much misunderstanding is from non-exposure," August said. "Nothing compared to standing in front of someone and staring at them, eye to eye – that's how to open your world. More often than not, you recognize the ways you are the same. Everyone has the same wants and needs."

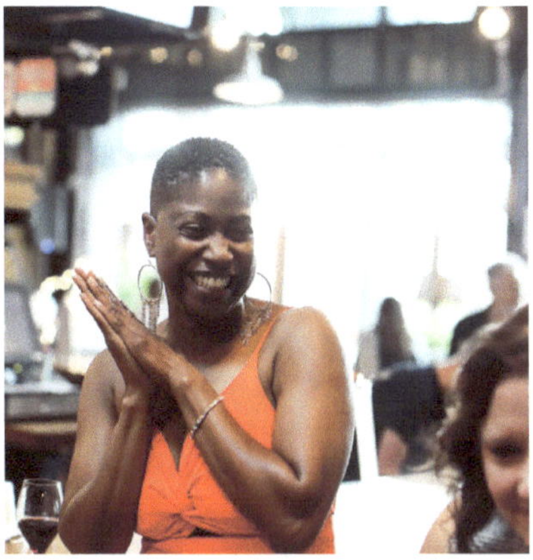

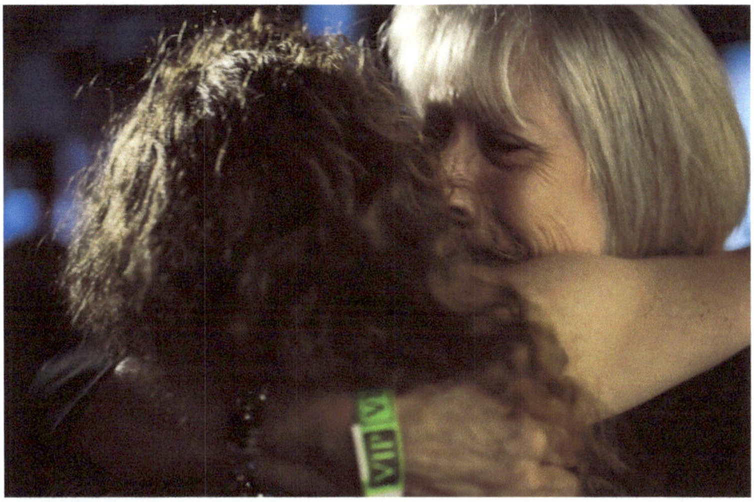

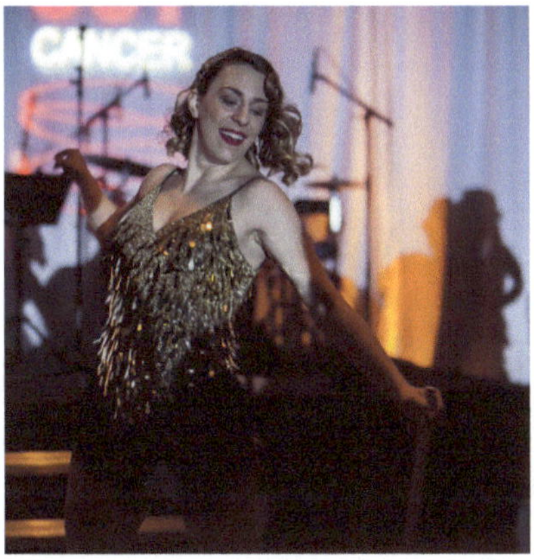

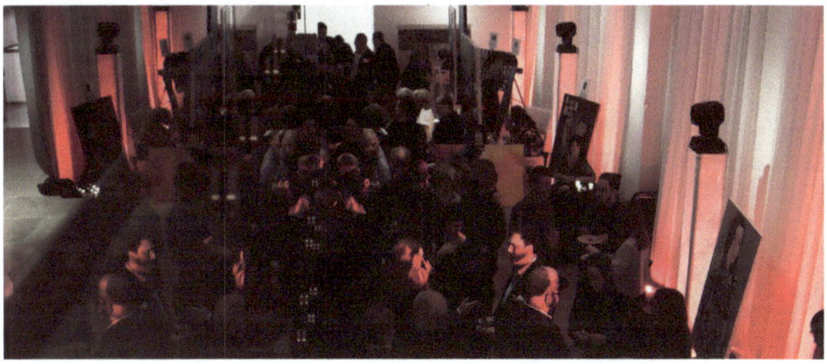

Another way Spree appreciates the Twist Out Cancer's international connections is through understanding cultures that are much different than her own. While mentoring an Inspiration in India, Spree learned how different the experience was from her own.

"I think more recently, I've come to see how different cancer is treated in other parts of the world and how important it is to bring more awareness."

Spree gives an example her mentee from India passed on.

"In India, there is a stigma around a woman's body and cancer," August said. "Twist Out Cancer is in a position to give a global voice to people who have dealt with cancer, and provide an opportunity for other people to speak up."

And that voice is spreading. The 2021 Brushes with Cancer virtual events had the most international participants of any year.

"Ten years ago, I didn't think I was going to get out of the hospital," Benn Shersher said. "To think that 140,000 people have been impacted by our work blows me away. I always said I wouldn't continue to do this if it stopped feeling good, and it has always felt good," Jenna said. "When you have nothing left to lose- dream big."

in memoriam

WE WOULD LIKE TO ACKNOWLEDGE AND HONOR OUR PAST BRUSHES WITH CANCER PARTICIPANTS WHO ARE NO LONGER WITH US PHYSICALLY, BUT ARE WITH US IN OUR HEARTS AND MINDS FOREVER.

Samantha Ainuddin
Terri Allister
Roy Arredondo
Ellen Bluestone
Jim Burke
Sunday Burquist
Samira Cooper
Chiara D'Agostino
Andrea Farquhar
Jackson Forssberg
Talia Gazlay
Mauren Gibbons Bole
Matt Gould
Noëlle Gray
Shawn Green
Brett Hoekema
Sophia Holland
Lauren Hubert Smoke
Tony Lollio
Patricia Lundstrom
Orit Maman Rada
Laura McCarty
Devon Messner
Mark Neil
Heather Newby
Alex Niles
Sian Oates
Kasey Passen
Danielle Peress
Amy Pizana
Stephanie Pratt
Dan Riordan
Maya Shany
Melissa Tang
Judy Waxman
Debra Yates

With Love & Gratitude

None of this would have been possible without the unwavering support of my family, friends and beloved Twist Out Cancer staff, board members and community. To David Shersher, the love of my life and my soul mate who has held my hand through every appointment, scan, and bump in the road for the last decade. To Noa and Lou, my miracle babies, who have shown me how far my heart is able to expand. To my parents Andrea and Eddie, and my sister Neely who have loved and supported me through every phase of my journey-thank you.

To Annie Kellner, Michele Kellner and Mark Kellner whose love and support has held me up during the most difficult of moments.

To Dan Hadad Aviad and Dan Fricker for being our chosen family.

To Sam Barsh and Jesse Palter for bringing music back into my life.

To Kasey Passen who may no longer walk beside me, but forever lives in my heart.

To Dr. Leo Gordon, Betsy Mitchell, Cecilia Gallo, Beth Young, and the entire team at Northwestern Hospital that saved my life. Words cannot express how grateful I am for your love, support, and care.

To Jeff Guerrero for the countless hours, creativity, and passion you have brought to bringing this book to life. I will never be able to properly thank you for all that you have done for us. To Joshua Taustein whose leadership and guidance helped give voice to so many. To Lindsay Patton who took the time to connect and dive deep into the lives of so many of our participants. To Kenny Lapins, Mardi Kaplan and Arlene Bonnet for your dedication and commitment to telling these stories.

To Amelia Hanrahan, my partner in crime who has helped to build Twist Out Cancer from the ground up.

To August Spree, Jacqueline Carmody, Jenna Koch, Ana Gordon, Dr. Lauren

Zaluda Rynar, Cai Fasse, and Mignon Dupepe who make up the Twist Out Cancer dream team.

To Andrew Edelston for his passion, leadership and commitment to strengthening Twist Out Cancer for the next decade.

To the extraordinary Twist Out Cancer Board; Emma Peck Block, Erin Johnson, Joelle Bilow, Stephanie Plein, Dr. Christian Squillante, Jon Goldberg, Howard Aaron, Jennifer Katz Margolis, Cynthia Beck, Danny Glick, Dr. Sharon Arffa, Kenny Lapins, Gudrun Wu Snyder, Jeffrey Guerrero, Dr. Martin Hogan, Mardi Kaplan, Kimberly Kass, Anna Feneis, Ella Hawk, Tanya Kertsman, Bari Murphy, Kara Thomas, and Shelby Zitelman. There is no better team to dream big with.

To Jonny Imerman, Ethan Zohn, Ann Altman, and Dr. Ann Feldman for being tremendous mentors and guides.

To Giorgia Lupi, Philip Cox, Ting Fang, Madeleine Garner, and the entire team at Pentagram for showcasing the intersection between pain and beauty.

To my darling Inti Velez, Dani Mancini and Iris Joval for immersing us in beauty.

To David Allen for taking a chance on us. You are magic!

To the entire Lombardo family for your generosity, leadership and LOVE.

To Iris Marreck, Steve Liska and Steve Juhasz for always making us look good.

To Katie Ashton for being the voice of reason.

To the Guenthner-Ashton Family and the Monieson Family for your continued support.

To the Coleman Foundation, Schusterman Foundation, Benjamin B. Green-Field Foundation and Smith Family Foundations for your belief in our mission and work.

To the inspirations who have bravely come forward and shared their stories and the artists that have generously shared their resources and gifts with us-we are in awe of you.

And to all those unnamed who played a role over the years—It has taken a village to arrive at this moment.

Here is to the next decade.

www.ingramcontent.com/pod-product-compliance
Lightning Source LLC
LaVergne TN
LVHW071239210926
848486LV00007B/303